GOD

&

BEATING CANCER AND
OTHER HEALTH CRISES

GOD

&

BEATING CANCER AND OTHER HEALTH CRISES

My Family, Faith & Fortitude

SHIRLEY VALENTINE

XULON PRESS

Xulon Press
2301 Lucien Way #415
Maitland, FL 32751
407.339.4217
www.xulonpress.com

Unless otherwise indicated, Scripture quotations taken from the King
James Version (KJV) – *public domain*.

Printed in the United States of America.

ISBN-13: 9781545612712

DEDICATION

This book is dedicated to all the beautiful people who have fought difficult battles with the dreaded disease called cancer. Some of us didn't make it through; some of us did; and some of us are still fighting for our lives. Either way, the battle is never over. We must always keep God in our prayers, praise His name first and, in time, He will answer. True spiritual believers of God tend to keep the faith of God in their hearts, minds and souls.

TABLE OF CONTENTS

PREFACE

In whole, this book is based primarily on my life experiences before, during and after my diagnosis with ovarian cancer. It's also based on the signs, symptoms and awareness of certain illnesses associated with my family's health history, i.e., ovarian cancer, breast cancer, lung cancer, uterine cancer, colon cancer, liver cancer, autism, thyroid disease, epilepsy & seizures, high blood pressure, stroke, heart attack, gout, gangrene, enlarged prostate, prostate cancer, shingles, lupus, arthritis, rheumatoid disease and diabetes.

The purpose of this book is to show others how focusing on what really matters in life can lead to peace as well as success. It also shows how utilizing Facebook as a tool for positive purposes was the magic key in bringing my family closer together. Through the grace of God and the love and support of family and friends, there's no way I could have made it.

I am honoring the people in my family who have made sacrifices for me and also by giving me the direction to fulfill my mother's dream of always putting "Family First." Thank you everyone for making my life what it is today. Whether you are here or afar, or just resting with the Lord, today I am honoring you ALL. *Amen.*

HONOREES

MY FAMILY TREE

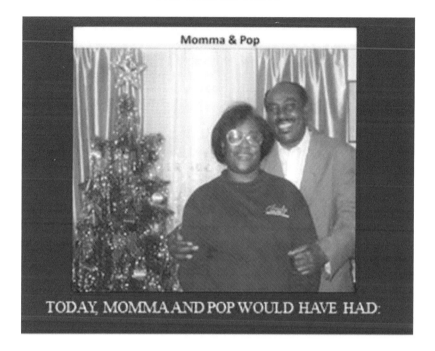

Momma & Pop

TODAY, MOMMA AND POP WOULD HAVE HAD:

8 CHILDREN

11 GRANDCHILDREN

15 GREAT GRANDCHILDREN

AND

4 GREAT GREAT-GRANDCHILDREN

WITH MORE ON THE WAY ...

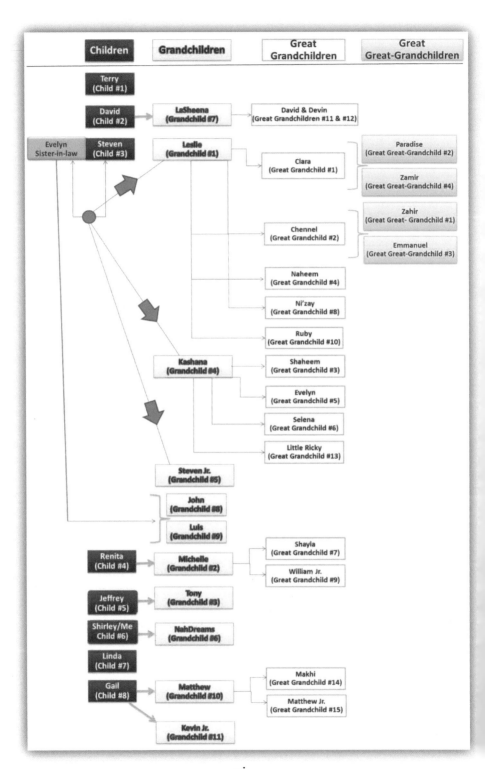

CHAPTER 1.   TIRED OF BEING TIRED

Over the years, Momma always said I was a good writer. But I never felt that way — everything I wrote came from the heart and always from good faith. Sometimes you gotta add a little sweet and sour to it — but it's all the same at the end of the day. I've always loved my poetry. I've always loved to write. I just never really did anything about it. So today, I am proud to reveal and happily share my poetry and prayers with you all.

> ## POETRY + PRAYER = PEACE
> ### &
> ## PEACE LIES WITHIN

The following poem was written and read to Momma prior to her demise. As I wrote it, I sensed a feeling of exhaustion, and then a big explosion. Why? I'm not sure, but I can only imagine what my feelings really were at that moment. Or, maybe my senses were telling me that someone else was actually tired of being tired. I wonder who that could've been — I should have known it was Momma. All the signs were there. I mean, I knew, hidden deeply inside, that it was actually her that was exhausted. Prior to her demise, Momma was more tired than anyone I knew, but she continued to keep going — non-stop and full-speed ahead!

I truly believe that God sent me this beautiful poem; kind of creating it as a red flag in regards to Momma's health. Oh Lord, I do remember how pleased she was to hear the poem, and insisted that it be published.

Tired of Being Tired

Apparition of the world's tribulations escalates higher
And because of this, the world can not be admired
Destruction, unemployment, hunger and pollution
Yesterday and today, another unsolved solution

I wish this image was only a test
And that the powers to be, take time to confess
That the problems are real, as real as can be
If we all work together, we can only achieve

Oil prices rising at an all time high
If this keeps up, no one will be able to buy
We need true people to take evaluations, surveys, you know
Everything of that nature to accommodate some dough

Maybe I need to back up, before I crack up
I don't want to give in before I rack up
On this truth, that I'm laying on you
And this terrible world that we all have reproduced

Standing alone would take more time
But working together will elevate our minds
To bring out the truth and work on ideas
That will help us resolve some of our worst nightmares

Shirley Valentine

I would ask myself, "Was this the way to begin my life over again? To do what I should have done in the first place? Give my life to God and live according to his ways? Today, I do have something to write about: "God & Beating Cancer And Other Health Crises: My Family, Faith & Fortitude." *Amen.*

CHAPTER 2.   THE BEGINNING

A. LIFE EXPERIENCES WITH MOMMA

Coming from humble beginnings, my parents have been together since their late teens and early twenties. Pop was always fortunate in landing promising jobs in the past so, after a long period of dedicated service with the Railroad, he eventually retired. Most of her life, Momma worked hard as a domestic housekeeper to support her family. Through their lives, they managed to raise eight children and eleven grandchildren. There were four boys and four girls, and I was the sixth child born.

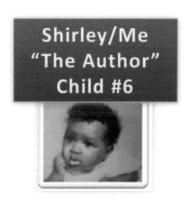

Shirley/Me "The Author" Child #6

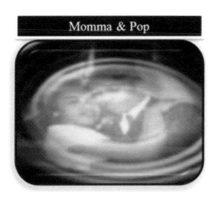

Momma & Pop

Growing up, we were a large family so our household was always busy. There was excitement everywhere we turned. Pop was supposed to be the leader, provider and loving father in our home, but sometimes he wasn't. Pop gave Momma a hard way to go with his compulsive drinking and gambling. When he drank, it would always lead to negative behavior: frivolous spending; gambling; lying; constant womanizing; etc. As long as I've known my Pop, he's always drank, smoked cigarettes, played poker, and contributed strenuous hurt to our family. Pop could be very hilarious at times, nevertheless, he lacked certain responsibilities and respect toward his family, especially toward Momma.

On occasional paydays, Pop would stay out overnight while spending his money unwisely. When he returned home, he wouldn't have a nickel in his pocket. Momma was always sick and tired of his nonsense. He rarely had enough funds to pay for a pack of cigarettes. At times, not being able to pay the utility bills or buy food was devastating to Momma. But she did what she needed to do to support her children.

Although we lived in a household growing up with both parents, I considered my Pop as a part-time deadbeat dad. Don't get me wrong, Pop was there at times, but not enough. He could have been more of a father to his children and more of a husband to his wife. People on the outside would always say how lucky we were to have a cool Pop, but they just didn't really know him. Yeah, he was very funny, and actually just as funny as Richard Pryor, and a colorful and outspoken man like Mohammad Ali. But his funny sense of humor was never the answer to paying any of the household bills. *Amen.*

On several occasions, if not more, Momma had to keep her head up and ask for support from her family. They, in turn, would help. However, due to the size of our family, sometimes we had to be separated as kids. The separation had to be very difficult for Momma, but family is all she knew. At least, we had the blessing of having family we could count on in difficult times. We, as kids, were very naïve as to what was actually going on — we were just having fun with our cousins. Of course, now that I'm an adult, I understand so much more than I did then. Momma had actually raised *nine* children instead of eight because Pop was the biggest kid of all. Now, ain't that something!

It was the late '60s in Brooklyn, New York and we lived in an apartment complex. I was approximately six or seven years of age, and playing with my two younger sisters, when something *terribly* went wrong. I accidentally stepped onto a book of matches and my mind went right into auto-mode. I gazed at the book of matches as if it were mesmerizing me. I then went over to my younger sisters and told them what I had found, but they were not really impressed. So, I figured I would go on and strike one of the matches from the book so that we all could see the beautiful flames. For some reason or another, the flames truly excited me.

Unfortunately, after striking the match, I didn't realize that I was standing directly over my bed when the match was lit. I held the lit match until it felt hot to my fingers and then, it fell right out of my hand, and onto the mattress. OMG! I was so in shock that I couldn't even move — I felt paralyzed as I didn't mean for that to happen. All I wanted to do was to see the rainbow of colors that the fire represented and in so doing, I had to strike a match — that's it. But now, everything was at a standstill — everything except the flames. The flames were spreading like wildflowers. I'm not quite certain what or how my little sisters were feeling but there was confusion on their faces and tears in their eyes. Once I saw their expressions, the shock wore off at that very moment and then Momma came rushing in. She was upset when she came into the room. And while she was trying to put out the fire, I was explaining what had occurred so, she got even more upset and immediately continued to put out the flames. I didn't exactly know what to do next, but my main concern was to help Momma put out the fire. And at that point, I was more in the way than anything. So, while Momma was filling a bucket with water, I was trying to quickly fill a cup with the same — while trying my best to help Momma extinguish the fire. When Momma noticed what I was doing, she kept yelling at me to drop everything and to get out! But we didn't want to leave Momma alone. Momma and the three of us eventually rushed outside of the apartment complex where it was safe, and the fire department did the rest.

No one was hurt or died from that fire. Thank God! As a young child, just the thought of *almost* hurting others made me feel miserable for a pretty long time.

Until this day, I still remember that incident so clearly — as if it happened just recently. Sometimes, I find it very difficult to forgive myself for creating such a tragedy. Although no one was hurt, we did lose everything, unfortunately. Our personal belongings meant the world to us, especially to Momma, but we couldn't salvage anything. Of course, as a child, I didn't understand the ramifications of what I had caused, but I do today.

I remember how Momma would remind me that she was planning on spanking me later for this incident. During this time, I was ill with the measles, so she decided to spank me after I recovered. Of course, I wanted the measles to last for a while — anything to avoid a spanking. But as time went by, and the measles eventually went away, Momma never did punish me with that spanking. She did, however, give me extra household chores to perform — and I'll take that over a spanking anytime. This photo was taken a little 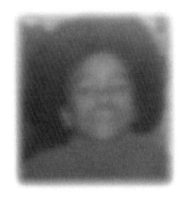 while after our family relocated to New York — shortly after the fire. I found it very hard to smile again after the incident in Brooklyn, but at times, I somehow managed to.

This is really the very first time I've actually mentioned this aloud to the world. I've always asked God to forgive me for the careless actions I caused that day, for I did not know better. And, I know He has forgiven me because He is a forgiving God. Who knows what our lives would've been like today if we didn't leave Brooklyn? By this time, Pop got a new job and our family had relocated to Queens, New York to continue living our lives again. Thank you God for not allowing physical harm to anyone during that time. *Amen.*

On one occasion during my teenage years, I worked under the summer youth program and was assigned to work at the neighborhood bus depot. In this position, along with other school kids, our duties included maintaining the cleanliness of the buses. The income made from this position enabled me to buy school clothing for the following school term.

On another occasion during my teenage years, I was employed as a dietary aide assistant at one of the local neighborhood hospitals. When my supervisor heard of my last name, she immediately connected my relationship to Momma as being her daughter. Interestingly enough, Momma and I had worked for the same hospital, in the same kitchen which was overseen by the same supervisor but at different times in our lives. When Momma worked for the hospital, she worked full time and had more responsibilities than me. I, along with other school kids, could only do but so much. As children, we worked under the summer youth program and received approximately $140.00 bi-weekly. My duties included: preparing meals/snacks; loading and distributing food trays; and maintaining the cleanliness of the kitchen and other duties assigned by the supervisor. Shopping for school clothing during this time was very exciting and rejuvenating for me. I was able to make my own money and pamper myself whenever I wanted to. What was so amazing was that every time the supervisor needed someone, she would call on me prior to the other school kids. Her reasoning in doing so was that I reminded her of how Momma was devoted and dedicated to her job and she believed that I could do the same.

When Momma found out about my summer job at the hospital, she couldn't believe it. Not only was the supervisor still working there, but so were other employees who were very close to Momma during her time of employment.

Over the years, Momma and I planned on being baptized, so finally, on November 12, 1989, we were both christened in a special ceremony at our

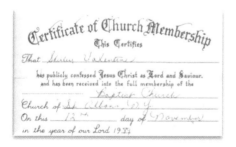

neighborhood community church. Our close family and friends were present to share in this sacred experience. We've always accepted Jesus Christ as our Lord and Savior, but felt deeply about having our baptism officially performed by a minister so that we may, in faith, honor Jesus and follow His way of life.

Immediately following the ceremony, we were presented with a copy of the Holy Bible to keep near and dear to our hearts. I will never forget how enchanted Momma and I felt after sharing a delightful and biblical moment together as a mother and daughter team. We also had the pleasure of becoming full members of our neighborhood community church. It was a long time coming for us, but we knew a change was going to come. *Amen.*

B. LIFE EXPERIENCES WITH POP

There was one particular occasion where I was so surprised to see my father, and that was at my high school graduation in June 1979. On this day, my parents were pleased and proud to see their daughter make it through twelve years of school. I was on my way and ready for the workforce. Corporations were already sending me job applications through the mail and I couldn't wait to complete and return them. *Amen.*

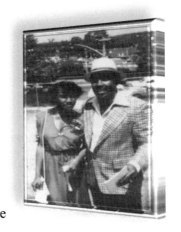

Pop, on one hand, was honored to see his daughter join the workforce. In his eyes, it was another income added into the household if I stayed. But on the other hand, I would have to live by his rules and his rules alone, with no exceptions. Now, tell me that wasn't being selfish. He also believed that once you become of age, which was 18, it was time to leave the nest. You could only stay at home with your parents if you were working or attending school. And that was the real deal in Pop's mind. Hey, like I said, sometimes he made a lot of us laugh, and sometimes he made us cry. I mean, afterall, over the years he's been wasting household funds, but yet continued to decide who stayed and entered into his home. But at this point, I began a new job and sadly moved out of my parents' house. This is where I began helping out my mother mentally and financially. But Pop kept that same mentality until the day he passed away because that's how he rolled.

At the beginning of each month, Momma would give Pop the household bills to place in the mail. He would soon after go to the bank to withdraw funds out of their account, knowing very well he was planning on spending the household funds frivolously. Then, after all of that, he'd have the nerve to return back home drunk and without any funds at all. This always made Momma sick, but there was nothing we could do but help pay the bills for her. I mean, thank goodness we were all grown up and able to assist by this time. I think it was part of Pop's plan — he didn't have to worry about paying for any bills because his children were now adults. He knew we wouldn't allow our mother to live without the basic utilities.

But in the meantime, while the family was expanding into the next generation, Pop doted over his grandchildren. Sometimes Pop had difficulties showing love, but he did devote a great deal of his time and energy to his grands, and loved them all unconditionally.

During the early stages of being grandparents, a number of memorable moments were spent at Momma and Pop's house. It was the early '80s, and on these occasions, the grandchildren were sharing moments of enjoying one of the simplest things in life – each other's company, while just sitting on the steps. It didn't make a difference whether it was winter or spring, because the grandchildren always enjoyed spending quality time at Momma's house. Leslie, Kashana and LaSheena were the first, fourth and seventh grandchildren born to Momma & Pop. *Amen.*

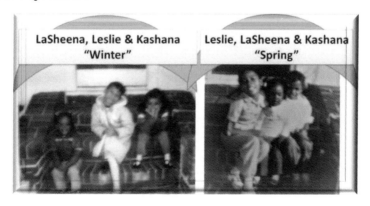

LaSheena, Leslie & Kashana
"Winter"

Leslie, LaSheena & Kashana
"Spring"

As time went by and the grands got older, Pop would continue to spend good times with them, and on this occasion, his granddaughter Michelle chose to do the teasing. She would tickle Pop until he couldn't take it anymore. LOL. Michelle was the second grandchild born to Momma & Pop.

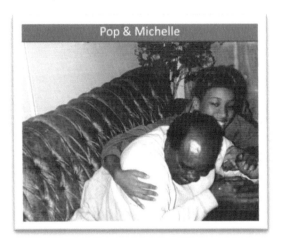

Pop & Michelle

When his grandson Matthew was born, Pop was a proud grandfather once again. Matthew was the next-to-the-last grandchild born.

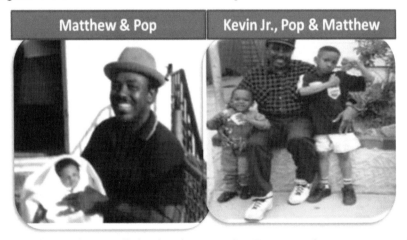

Matthew & Pop | Kevin Jr., Pop & Matthew

And Matthew's little brother Kevin Jr. was the youngest of the grandchildren and Pop, spoiled both these guys altogether. Pop would walk with these two to the corner store to purchase them some goodies. Kevin loved the attention and would follow his grandpa just about anywhere, whereas Matthew always believed that the goodies would make him stronger. LOL. Bless their little hearts. *Amen.*

Pop loved spending quality time with his other grandson as well. Steven Jr. was his pride and joy and Pop took honor in taking this photo with him. Pop at times, would talk to Steven Jr. about life in general, and all the possibilities it had to offer — man-to-man kind of stuff. Of course, whenever I would hear the advice Pop would give, I had no other option but to laugh. Pop had a lot of good in him, and sometimes gave out good advice; however, he didn't provide the same type of behavior to his own children. He was pretty strict with us and knocked us around every once in a while to show who was the boss. He always said that his father was strict on him and his siblings and that's why he was so strict with us. It was going to be his way, or the highway and that was that. But when the grandchildren came along and we all were adults, Pop slowed down a great deal with the punishments. I guess there are some things in life that will make a person change somewhat.

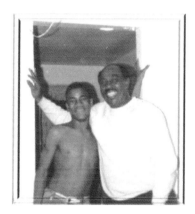

Pop loved to read the *New York Daily News* and also listened to the news on TV. However, at times, he would hear something totally different. Although he wore a hearing aid, he was proud to be hearing again, but he really wasn't hearing correctly.   Sometimes, when watching and listening to the news, Pop would complain about the violence going on in the world. But then, Momma would take notice and innocently correct him, but he would get upset and continue to tell the same story anyway.

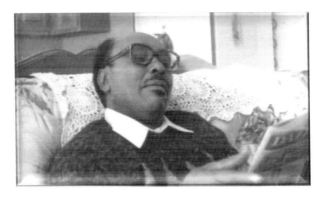

As time went by, his hearing worsened and he refused to take any further action to resolve the problem. And then, there were times when you would raise your voice to make certain he heard you, and he would then tell you to stop shouting. Sometimes we just didn't know what to think. According to Pop, he hears what he wants to hear and that was that.

Pop also enjoyed purchasing ice cream from the Mister Softee truck and shared it with the entire family. Sometimes he would need an ice cream cone tray to hold the ice cream because he always seemed to buy too much of it. At times, the ice cream would quickly melt prior to us even receiving it, but that didn't stop us from enjoying and appreciating the treats. Pop was very generous when it came to his favorite desserts and this was one we all enjoyed as a family. *Amen.*

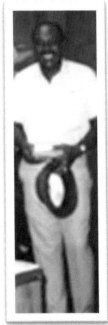

Over 20 years of dedicated service with the Railroad, Pop was fortunate to retire at the early age of 62. It was the end of the line for Pop because he finally achieved his most rewarding goal. After receiving his retirement plaque, he was so excited that he graciously thanked everyone and then quickly hightailed it back home to show it off. This was a very unique and special day for Pop and we all were very proud of him.

Unfortunately, Pop was diagnosed with a light stroke, and, in his later years, an enlarged prostate. He had to be hospitalized for a short while, but endured a great deal of pain and suffering while going through this process. Through the grace of God and the strength of our family, he was able to pull through. *Amen.*

Prior to Momma's death, husband Ed and I had accompanied Pop to a car dealership in Jamaica, Queens. Pop wanted our opinion about purchasing a van he had his eye on for a while, so Ed and I were more than delighted to assist. When we arrived to the dealership's office, we were led outside to the car lot to see the actual van. Once approached, it appeared to be in pretty decent shape for a *used* van. And, when we looked inside, it was very spacious and held a total of six passengers. The entertainment center included a mini TV set, VCR/DVD player and two sets of surround sound speakers.

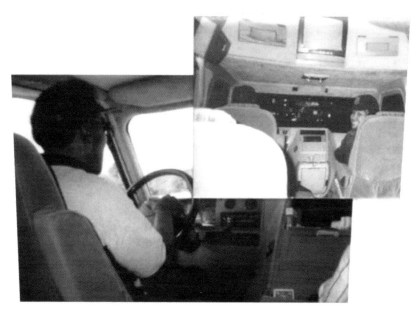

If anybody rode side-by-side with Pop on trips to Atlantic City, it would've been me. Front row seat and passenger side was always my choice.

You couldn't tell me anything. The middle two seats had the capability of leaning like a recliner for better comfort. The backseat converted into a bed or folded upright for extra seating. I loved treating Pop and Momma on special occasions. Sometimes it was just because ... and that's how I rolled.

Since the van was mainly for transportation to and from Atlantic City, we decided to give it a name. The new name was now called "The AC Van" and I enjoyed every moment in it. Hey, Pop may have been a complicated man, but he was still a man, and a funny one at that! *Amen.*

Immediately following Momma's death, Pop was distraught and very confused, but we tried to minimize some of his depression with fun and laughter. That, of course, wasn't always the answer though — sometimes when couples have committed a great number of years together, and one passes on, the other usually has a difficult time surviving without the other. And, although Pop was surrounded by a number of family and friends on a daily basis, he was still actually lonely. His family could fulfill only some of his needs. His and Momma's relationship may have been rocky over the years, but it was theirs nonetheless. The deep passion and long lifetime of togetherness that was built with Momma, could never be shared with anyone else. So, as time went by, Pop was getting increasingly weary and gloomy, while at the same time, missing Momma in the worse way. This of course, was a heavy burden on Pop, as his life no longer had the same meaning!

He always said if he had to go, let it be in Atlantic City because that was his favorite place to be. Folks thought Pop was just running his mouth off as usual, but at the end of the day, he meant every word. And ironically, that's exactly where he passed away. Sorrowfully, on March 5, 2007, and almost three years since Momma's death, Pop did pass away in Atlantic City, just like he had preferred.

Pop liked to often use popular quotes, and then share these quotes with the world. He was like social media, but an actual walking/human Facebook post and, posting the same posts every single day. That was Pop. LOL. It wasn't necessarily *what* he said, but *how* he would say it. His response for just about everything always ended with one of the following terms: *"I'm a bad man," "I can't stand nothing," "Tell your story walking," "Just look at all the fun we had," "Ya'll gonna make me lose my mind, up in here, up in here,"* and finally, his favorite: *"What about me?"* Pop was definitely a funny character at heart.

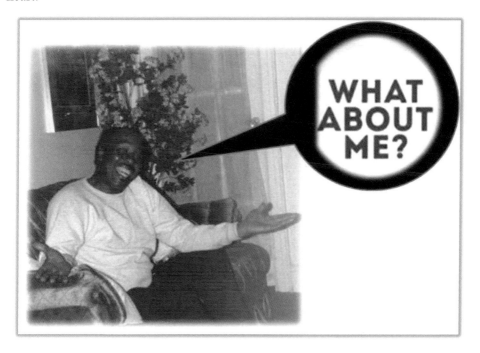

At least I can say, I had a lot of fun and good laughs with my Pop over the years and through all these crazy and ridiculous memories, he'll remain alive in me. And that said, I will always love and miss him dearly, despite his imperfections. He was my father and that will never change, and I will never doubt his love for me. May you rest in peace Pop. *Amen.*

CHAPTER 3.   YEARNING FOR MOM

It was June 13th, 2004, and sadly, Momma's last day on this earth. Through her complicated and conflicted life she had managed to raise a very large family. Although she may have had some help from my Pop — believe me — it wasn't much at all, Pop did his thing and didn't care at times who got hurt. But Momma always looked out for us. I've always said:

"Remember, no one is going to love you in this world more than God and your Momma."

Momma and Pop are seen here, in 1958, with their first four children. My family looked amazing and probably could've made it in the modelling business. LOL. And although their hands were full with these four, that didn't stop them from creating another four. *Amen.*

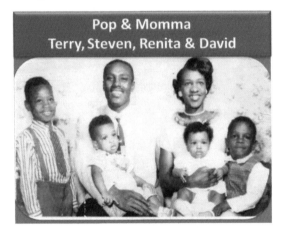

Pop & Momma
Terry, Steven, Renita & David

Together with my Pop, Momma gave birth to four boys and four girls by the age of 30. She molded herself to become the best wife and mother ever.

During the late '60s, and also my childhood years, at times, I used to accompany Momma to work. Momma would perform domestic duties and had to travel on a few buses to get there. I would help her clean houses, go grocery shopping and prepare meals for the sick and elderly. I've always loved going to work with Momma, because that gave me the opportunity to spend quality time with her. As busy as she was with the rest of the family, this was going to be my time — and my time only. I didn't always think she had the best job in the world, but I've always respected her for taking care of her family. You see, Momma may not have acquired much education in her lifetime, but she did, however, possess qualities that only a loving mother would have toward her family. *Amen.*

I recall one incident which occurred on a school day. Gail, Linda and myself, all attended the same elementary school and would walk home on our lunch break to share it with Momma. But on this day, when we knocked on the door, there was no response. We walked around the house to try to look inside the windows, but couldn't find anything out of the ordinary. We therefore, sat on the steps of our house for a short while when our neighbors from across the street noticed our confusion. They found it strange that we were sitting outside in the middle of a school day, so they came over to ask if everything was all right. I kindly explained to them how we came home for lunch but Momma wasn't home or at least, not responding. The neighbors knocked on the door as well, but when they didn't get a response either, they generously welcomed us into their home to provide lunch, until we heard from Momma. We were so delighted and blessed to have such good neighbors and hoped everything was fine with Momma.

Shortly after, while we were still eating our lunch at the neighbor's, Momma had arrived home. The neighbors took notice of Momma's arrival and made certain to inform her of our location. She was so happy to hear it and was very apologetic for inconveniencing them in any way. But they wouldn't have it and assured Momma that it was not a problem at all. Momma's dilemma was that she was running late because she had to stop off at the grocery store prior to heading back home. She wanted to make certain that we, her children, were provided with the proper vitamins and nutrients for the remainder of the week. But, when she got to the grocery store, she had no idea it would be overly crowded and so, the shopping took a little longer than usual. And then, once she bought all her groceries, she had to actually take two buses home, while at the same time, carry these full bags of groceries. There was no stopping Momma when it came to feeding her family though — she wasn't giving up at all. And, once we graciously completed eating our lunch at the neighbors, we had a few more minutes remaining to spend with Momma. Every second of every minute was enjoyed with Momma, and by the end of our lunch period, we returned back to school, and Momma, back to work. *Amen.*

But as we grew and matured to become the responsible adults our parents wished for, we created our own families, and the new generation began.

Over the years, Momma has done so much for us, especially with help in raising our children. Fortunately, we were able to talk Momma into becoming a stay-at-home mom and receive pay for her dedicated services. Momma thought this was a good idea and therefore agreed. By this time, her daughters were all working and were capable of providing her with a steady income. Also, the thought of actually returning to riding on buses and performing domestic housecleaning didn't sound appealing at all to Momma. In fact, it never did. In any event, we were grateful that Momma was now home and not on those mean streets of New York anymore. *Amen.*

In order to keep up with the next generation, Momma had to juggle her way in life. After getting him to sleep, Momma placed her grandson, Steven Jr., down for a more relaxing rest, and then slid over to the other side of the sofa to show some love to her other grandson and my only child, NahDreams. Mind you, NahDreams was just born and Steven Jr. was only seven months older than he, and even today, they remain close and continue to share fond memories together.

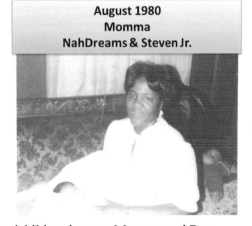

August 1980
Momma
NahDreams & Steven Jr.

These guys were the fifth and sixth grandchildren born to Momma and Pop.

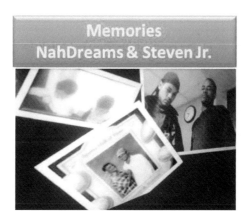

Momma was constantly busy with her loving and energetic grandchildren. In this picture, there are seven of eleven grandchildren born and the other four (John, Luis, Matthew and Kevin) hadn't been born yet.

Early '80

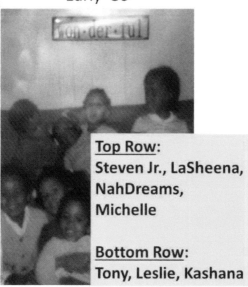

Top Row:
Steven Jr., LaSheena, NahDreams, Michelle

Bottom Row:
Tony, Leslie, Kashana

Pop wasn't the only one having fun, Momma enjoyed going out and having some fun as well — she just didn't have as much. If there was any way I could make Momma smile, I would take every opportunity in doing so. So, my sisters and I would treat Momma to occasional breakfasts or lunches at IHOP or take her on trips to Miami.

It was the late '80s and my sisters and I had decided to take Momma and the kids on a trip to Florida to explore the other side of the coast. It was a beautiful time when the family enjoyed each other's company. But, no matter where we were, Momma always had something on her mind!

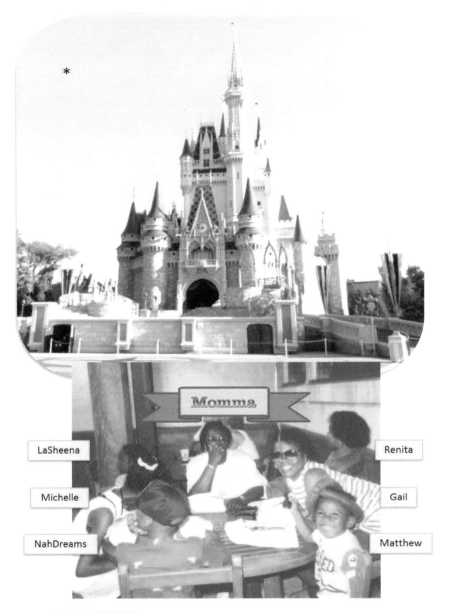

* http://hypeorlando-prod.s3.amazonaws.com/in-the-shadow-of-the-mouse/wp-content/uploads/sites/62/2014/04/temp41.jpg

Goofy & Me	Michelle

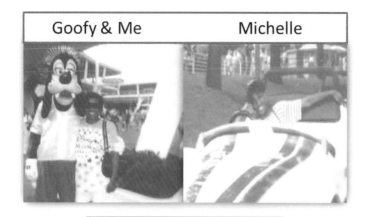

Momma, Gail & Renita

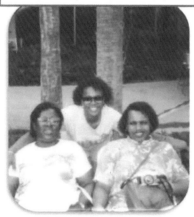

Matthew & Gail	Me & LaSheena

Matthew, NahDreams, Gail & LaSheena

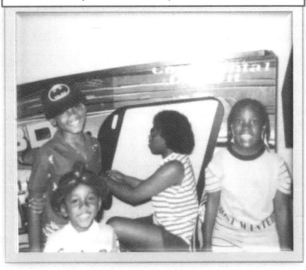

NahDreams, Michelle & Goofy

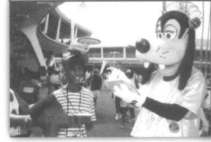

LaSheena, Matthew & NahDreams

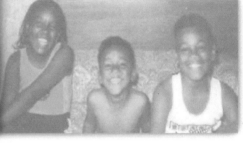

Michelle & Renita

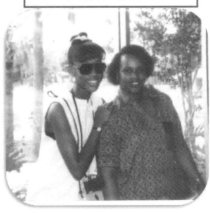

We would also treat Momma to Atlantic City for good times. And, when not in Atlantic City, we would do things like play her favorite board games such as checkers and bingo with her to pass the time.

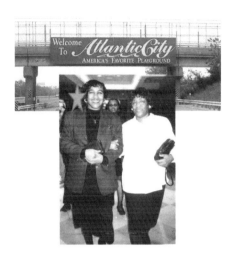

My sisters and I would accompany Momma to church functions and sometimes would participate in the activities. We took pride in singing in the choir, directing the children's choir, performing in the Women's Day event as well as other events. Interacting with the church members was a tremendous blessing as well.

During NahDreams' elementary school days, Momma was also active in attending special functions. In this picture, NahDreams was awarded a

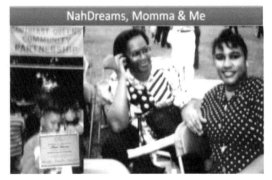

Certificate of Appreciation for his recognition of services to the Southeast Queens Community Center. We were all proud because NahDreams was able to achieve such a wonderful accomplishment in his life. Along with others, goals were made and growing up to become better individuals was one of Momma's most precious dreams for her grandchildren.

It was the mid '90s and Christmas time in Queens at Momma's house. This was the final picture taken of the grandchildren prior to Momma's demise. Although you kids enjoyed the holiday season, your faces were surely expressing something different.

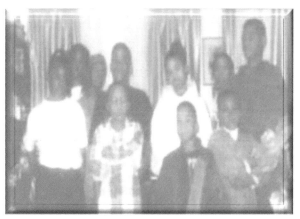

Prior to Momma's demise, she was diagnosed with thyroid disease, a light stroke, gout, high blood pressure, and eventually suffered a heart attack. Over the years, she was able to get through the removal of a non-cancerous tumor as well as a triple by-pass operation. Thank you God.

However, as time went by, these sicknesses made her extremely weak and helpless. The predators continued to feed off of her though. Constant visits, awaiting great meals and begging for money was a daily routine in our household. No one took into consideration that she used every bone and muscle in her weak body to please them.

The death of Momma broke the link to the entire family. She was very ill — consuming approximately a dozen medications on a daily basis which enabled her to go on as long as she did. Her demise was inevitable, though — especially the way the family saw her through their selfish eyes. They practically believed she was immortal, and therefore would always be there for them. I could see the weight on her shoulders bringing her down, but I couldn't convince the family to take direct notice. Trying desperately to relieve some of her pressures, and not succeeding, eventually took a toll on me.

I believe her death was caused from family stress and tension. In hindsight, they didn't actually realize the pain and suffering that they had caused her and they unwittingly ignored the signs. Momma found it very difficult to say the word "No". To her, that word symbolized her incapability of helping out her family no matter what the consequences were. And, therefore, she would say whatever it took to put a smile on our faces and to give us what we needed. She would pray for us when we really 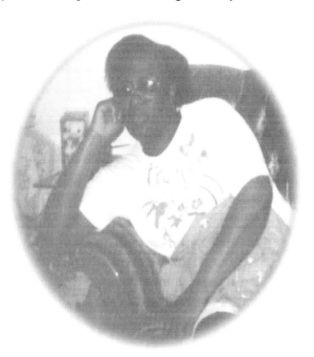 needed to pray for ourselves. But when she would comfort us, she was actually comforting herself. Momma was a strong individual who took pride in everything she ever accomplished, and, at the end of her life, her family didn't learn a thing.

For many years, she was a former dedicated Usher and Leader to the Women's Group at her Baptist Church. She was a loyal and devoted member since the late '80s and believed in helping her fellow members unconditionally.

But whether it was for love, attention, feeding the hungry, prayer or just good old fashion conversation, friends and family members knew where to turn. Momma provided just about anything an individual could ever ask for in order to make their day brighter.

However, everyone refused to hear her cries. Maybe they really couldn't because of her beautiful smile. On many occasions, when she did smile, she was actually crying within. But, at times, her body language and certain gestures told the real truth about the way she felt at a given moment. She was a dedicated wife, the master of motherhood, a treasured gift to her grandchildren, and the most beloved person in our household. She was especially an inspiration to me!

Now that she's gone, we reach for her and realize that she is no longer there. I gaze at her picture every day and wonder if there was anything possible I could have done to save her. But in retrospect, she had already been saved. She was now with Jesus Christ, her Lord and Savior. But when she was here on this earth, I made it a personal point to make her happy.

Momma was kind, generous, thoughtful, sweet and, most of all, forgiving. She would always give people the benefit of a doubt, despite their track record. She believed that if someone could change for the worse, then they could definitely change for the better.

Always putting herself last, she allowed certain individuals to take advantage of her kindness. They were predators. They consistently came into her life, using and abusing her health and generosity and demonstrating greed and selfishness. She would accept their selfish ways and cling onto the goodness within them. Being unselfish was always Momma's way. *Amen.*

Eventually, all of the anguish she experienced over the years took a toll on her, both mentally and physically. But she was determined to continue to attend church and pray on a daily basis. This alone would relieve some of her most deepest pressures.

In any event, Momma honestly believed that when you do honest work, you are working for the Lord. And performing her tasks as an usher at our community church was working for the Lord. That's exactly how Momma felt.

I recall clearly, in May of 2004, our church held a special event in honor of Women's Day where Momma and others were being honored. Momma thrived and took pride in establishing the leadership role of the Women's Day — Group #3 at our community church.

For this special occasion, Momma had to actually coerce some of the family members into participating in the event *together*. She insisted that this would be the last Women's Day event she would be attending. We would tell Momma to not speak in that manner and to instead always think positive. But she didn't pay any attention to us. The family was always aware of Momma's poor health condition (and sometimes I wonder if we really knew everything about it). Afterall, Momma was good at keeping some family secrets. Maybe there's more to the story than meets the eye. Who knows?

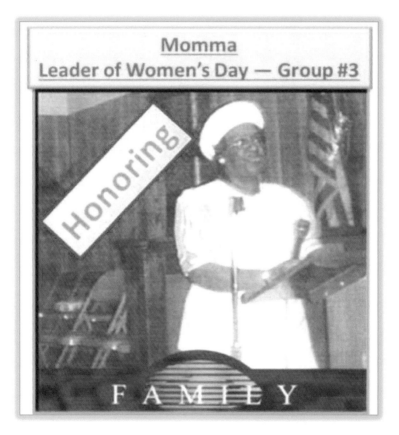

I think about her on a regular basis and she'll always be with me. So the following year, I developed the courage to write and publish a poem in honor of Momma:

Yearning for Mom

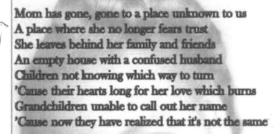

Mom has gone, gone to a place unknown to us
A place where she no longer fears trust
She leaves behind her family and friends
An empty house with a confused husband
Children not knowing which way to turn
'Cause their hearts long for her love which burns
Grandchildren unable to call out her name
'Cause now they have realized that it's not the same

Yearning for Mom, over and over again
Her friends, her fellow church members and the rest
of her kin
We're praying and believing that it was her time
That she has earned her wings and is no longer
confined
Free from the agony and pain she has suffered
Free from the anguished dissolution that was
discovered

Oh, how we yearn, we yearn for her love
We yearn for her spirit and we yearn for her hugs
Her courage, her strength and her warm embrace
Her kiss, her smile and her cheerful face
We yearn for her, day in and day out
But we will never forget, the love she gave throughout

Shirley Valentine
Copyright ©2005

I dedicated this poem in remembrance of a very special lady, Momma. She departed this life on Sunday, June 13, 2004, and will be forever loved and missed. Throughout my lifetime, she has given me the inspiration and motivation to express myself by writing poetry. I will always be indebted to her for her loyalty and strength in raising a large family. Her dedication to our family has taken me to a totally different level in life. It has taught me to continue her journey in bringing our family closer together.

CHAPTER 4.   MY FIRST WORD PROCESSING COMPUTER

Back in those days, the electric typewriter was an electromechanical machine utilized in mainstream offices all over the world. However, when the '80s approached, I was bored using the typewriter, and computers ushered in a whole new era. Due to the increase in the workload, a computer was essential for our department at that time. My boss also saw future potential in me and decided to do something about it. So, when she suggested we purchase a computer for

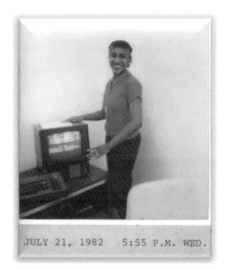

JULY 21, 1982   5:55 P.M. WED.

the office, I was excited and couldn't wait for management to place the order. However, for this dream to become a reality, I would have to teach the functions and features of the software to myself. Who was I to complain? I couldn't, because the company was considerate enough to provide training manuals to make my self-training easier. I also thought about the added capability I'd have in completing work in a more timely

fashion which would lead to more time for self-training. Therefore, I agreed to the terms and conditions, and the new computer was ordered for the office.

Several months later, I became knowledgeable with the software and functions, and my opportunities were endless. I found the entire training process to be quite challenging, yet exhilarating. In order to bring my speed and accuracy up to top-notch perfection, I would find interesting and fun ways of challenging myself. This was one of the most gratifying experiences — showing others the skills I had happily acquired. With the new computer, I managed to get the completion of the workload down to half the time. Now, time was allowed for other administrative duties in the office. I also had the opportunity to work with so many beautiful people who taught me, at an early age, how to succeed professionally. I'll never forget how they would complement me on how motivated I was at such an early age.

I would like to thank you all for your teachings as well as your friendship. God bless.

As days turned into weeks, and weeks into months, and the years accumulated, my professional skills advanced into a leadership position. By the late '80s, I was honored to accept the role as supervisor and lead the department into the right direction.

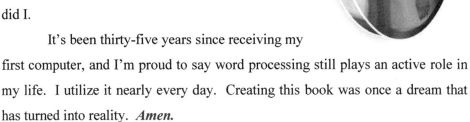

I was elated about obtaining a position where I could wake up every morning and feel proud to go to work. However, my personal life was another matter. Sometimes, situations were complicated, but in any event, life went on. And so did I.

It's been thirty-five years since receiving my first computer, and I'm proud to say word processing still plays an active role in my life. I utilize it nearly every day. Creating this book was once a dream that has turned into reality. *Amen.*

CHAPTER 5.   THE MOVE

One of my favorite television series today is Curtis "50 Cent" Jackson's "Power." The show is a mad success and the theme song is astounding. The show is based on high crime in the Big Apple, New York City, and my hometown. As 50 Cent would say:

> "It's a big rich town. I just come from the poorest part. Bright
> lights, city lights I got to make it. This is where it goes down."

The only problem: I didn't make it in New York City. I made it in South Carolina. But it really didn't matter because, through the grace of God, I made it. *Amen.*

My life story begins in December 1961 where I was raised in New York City. Eventually, upon reaching adulthood, I was employed for many years as a word processor/supervisor for several corporate law firms as well as investment banks and other institutions.

Unfortunately, due to 9/11 and the stagnated economy, my employment in 2009 was in jeopardy and was eventually terminated. But prior to terminating me, management decided to let the others go first — and just like me, we were called into the conference room one-by-one, like little Indians. And just like a chief — I was the last of the Mohicans. Prior to our termination, we did sense the gray clouds lingering over our jobs but realistically couldn't do anything about it. The pain from watching the folks you love and admire, to:

- receiving a phone call to meet in a conference room without explanation;
- shortly returning back to the word processing center to clean out your desk and personal matters; and then
- being escorted out the building by security

was a lot to handle.

This wasn't exactly my idea of any teamwork at all. It was only predictable for management to handle the situation in this manner. It appeared to me that "teamwork" suited their own corporate needs and not the needs of the staff.

As time went by, I continuously searched for employment in New York, but to no avail. There just wasn't any available word processing work at the time. While people were constantly being laid off, companies were constantly downsizing and outsourcing. There was no time to feel sorry for yourself or the situation at hand as it was time to move on. Besides, with the rise in unemployment, it was just a matter of time before the majority of our jobs were sacrificed! So, as for me and my family, we _sadly_ had to make the decision to relocate to South Carolina.

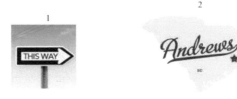

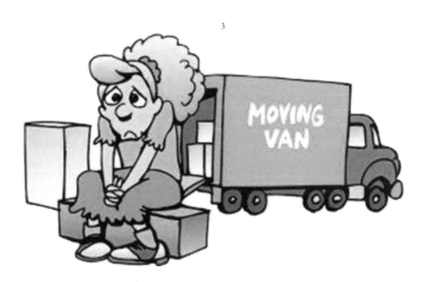

[1] http://spearmarketing.com/blog/wp-content/uploads/2011/08/this-way-sign.jpg
[2] http://townmapsusa.com/images/maps/map_of_andrews_sc.jpg
[3] https://encrypted-tbn3.gstatic.com/images?q=tbn:ANd9GcQ_mbX5G76s9aifa2BoiHUDu915P1_o1_77Vp0wyC2cTiCUJD9E

And, after all these years, I've been living as a "Native New Yorker" (one of my favorite songs):

> Runnin' pretty, New York City girl
> Twenty-five, thirty-five
> Hello baby, New York City girl
>
> You grew up riding the subways running with people
> Up in Harlem, down on Broadway
> You're no tramp but you're no lady talkin' that street talk
> You're the heart and soul of New York City
>
> And love, love is just a passing word
> It's the thought you had in a taxi cab
> That got left on the curb
> When he dropped you off at East 83rd
>
> You're a native New Yorker
> You should know the score by now
> You're a native New Yorker

Well, here we were in South Carolina now, and it was just as hard finding work here as it was in New York. I guess a "global change" is actually a global change. I just refused to accept how all of our lives would be affected by this drastic change in the economy.

Although we had only lived in the South for a couple of months now, my heart was missing my family and friends and the desire to return to New York kept haunting me. Eventually, I had to let that idea go because my heart was saying one thing, but my pocketbook was saying another.

A little while later, I did find part-time employment but after a couple of failed jobs, I settled as a cook/dishwasher for a fast food restaurant that paid minimum wage. I wasn't really concerned with the type or pay of the job; my intent was to do my best so that I could pay my household bills.

Almost two years passed and I was feeling fine and looking great — at least I thought. Then, unbeknownst to me at the time, my life would dramatically change forever.

This is a true story about my struggle with ovarian cancer and how I survived this fight through the grace of God and with the love and support of my family and friends. *Amen.*

CHAPTER 6.   LAST DAY OF WORK — PRIOR TO DIAGNOSIS / VALENTINE'S DAY / FEBRUARY 14, 2014

Going to work on this particular day wasn't usually an option for me, since no work = no pay. That's how it goes. So I did what I had to do and went to work that evening. It was my last night of work when I felt something just wasn't right. I worked very hard as a cook/dishwasher in the kitchen of a fast food restaurant in South Carolina. I was employed there for less than two years and never had a problem with job performance.

It was a couple of hours until closing when I realized we ran out of potato wedges. Well, time to trot on over to the supply room and pick up a box of potatoes, I thought. However, when I went to raise the box, the lower right back side of my stomach area began to throb in horrific pain. I immediately dropped the bag of potatoes to the floor and quickly ran back into the kitchen to inform my co-worker and dear friend Tiffany who was working with me that evening. She took action right away and made certain that I would stop working immediately. Tiffany demanded that I sit down, relax and not lift a finger for the remainder of the night, to which I agreed. Who knows what could have happened if I didn't stop working that night. And because of her loyal dedication and quick actions, she may have saved a dear friend's life — mine. Thanks for making the right choice that night, Tiffany. You are my Angel. *God bless.*

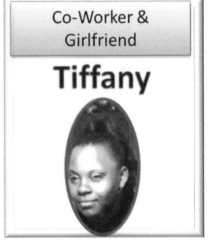

Eventually, within the next two hours, the shift was over. When I returned home, I mentioned the unfortunate mishap to my husband and older sister. They both agreed that I go directly to the hospital the following morning.

THANK GOD I DID. Even at that point I didn't really realize the severity of my condition, but I did feel something just wasn't right.

Up until this point, the kitchen was overly heated and very often unbearable to work in. I still don't know how I lasted as long as I did. But I do know that I prayed just about everyday for God to help me to find a way out of that kitchen. Through the grace of God, a way was found — God's way! And at the end of the day, it was still Valentine's Day...

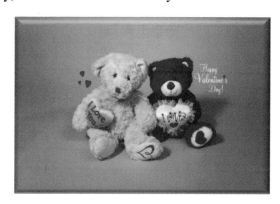

CHAPTER 7.   DIAGNOSED IN FEBRUARY 2014
& MCLEOD'S MEDICAL TEAM

After testing at Williamsburg Regional Hospital in Kingstree, South Carolina, a large growth was found in my abdominal area. Shortly thereafter, I was transferred to McLeod Regional Medical Center in Florence, South Carolina for additional testing and procedures.

After another several rounds of testing at McLeod Regional Medical Center, a large tumor was confirmed in the abdomen. Options for treatment were discussed followed by tumor removal by Dr. John Chapman, OB/GYN. Unfortunately, the tumor was found to be malignant, staged, and was then treated by Dr. James C.H. Smith, Oncologist, and his Associates at McLeod's Cancer Treatment & Research Center.

And here I was thinking, after all of these months, how proud I was of myself for losing the weight that I wasn't even trying to lose. I was proud and you couldn't tell me anything — I just knew surely that slaving in a hot kitchen

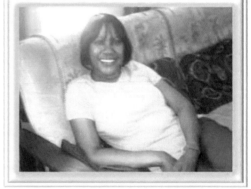

and perspiring all day was the cause of my rapid weight loss. My weight went from 185 lbs. down to 142 lbs. in a matter of months. This was completely unplanned, and, in hindsight, it was one of the red flags I failed to recognize.

Some of the symptoms I noticed included: the dramatic weight loss, fewer visits to the bathroom, hardly any appetite, and the consistent throbbing pain on the lower-right back side of my stomach. *Thank God for those RED FLAGS.*

I felt scared but strong, all at the same time. My entire intake on this ordeal — with all the illnesses in my family, ovarian cancer wasn't actually on my list. I was emotionally dealing with a disease I had no knowledge of. But, my family's strength in getting through tough times has encouraged me to fight this battle right to the end. And, with a nursing staff at McLeod to occasionally stop by to lift my spirits with prayers and kind words, I couldn't lose.

I have great respect and honor for the doctors who I believe saved my life. With all the MRIs, CT Scans and blood work involved, I really didn't care because all I wanted was to have these cancer cells removed from my beautiful body. But either way you look at it, it was time for surgery, and on the day of February 16, 2014, I was prepped and ready to go!

After having the malignant ovarian tumor removed, I returned to my hospital room for about one week to recover. During this period, I had a lot of time to think and realized that He has spoken, and I — I had another chance at life. I also realized that everything in life does have a purpose, and getting back on my feet was mine. *Amen.*

From the moment I heard my diagnosis until the end of my hospital stay, I don't think I had a decent night's sleep. My husband Ed would remind me on several occasions how strong I was because through it all, my attitude remained positive. *Amen.*

Pretty hard to explain how you're supposed to feel when you think your life is being cut short. I know my first thought was "no, I didn't hear what I think I heard" and then thinking to myself, "you're speechless 'cause you're really in shock". But then, as the seconds turn into minutes — you catch on and then reality kicks in — like a ton of bricks. But that wasn't quite the case — Although I was informed that I was in Stage IIIC with ovarian cancer, there was still hope for me. Thanks, Dr. Smith, for lifting my spirits — I needed that. Nothing was left to say after the removal of the cancerous tumor, except ask, "What's the next step?" And after discussing my options, we decided to go with "Chemotherapy". *Amen.*

During my stay, my sister Gail would come to visit and assist in filling out paperwork needed for the hospital. The hospital staff along with outside support organizations would also visit to see if I needed any professional counseling, support groups or other resources to help with my recovery process.

The nursing staff was very mindful and considerate of my needs and made certain that if any discomfort occurred, they would handle it immediately. If you wanted the staff to pray or sing with you, they would. If you needed one of them to listen to your jokes, they would do that too. I recall one time when a nurse was drawing blood and noticed that I was a little nervous. She heard me praying and then actually prayed with me. Prayer was my way of distracting from the thought of receiving the actual shot. I didn't mind needles so much, I just didn't have any remaining "good" blood vessels to tend with. So, after a couple of unsuccessful tries in the arm, we decided to take from the back of the hand. I wasn't quite keen on this idea either, but did what I had to do and, going forward, a number of my visits included drawing blood from the back of my hand. But it really didn't matter. Either way, the nursing staff here at McLeod made you feel right at home. They are true to their patients! God Bless Them All. *Amen.*

MCLEOD'S MEDICAL TEAM

McLeod Regional Medical Center /
McLeod Center for Cancer Treatment & Research
in Florence, South Carolina
has a WONDERFUL Medical Team:

Dr. John Chapman   Dr. James C.H. Smith
OB/GYN   Oncologist

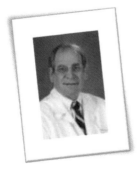   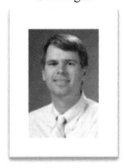

Cancer Report 2015[4]

Annually, the McLeod Center for Cancer Treatment & Research publishes a Cancer Report designed to build community awareness of our cancer services. The 2015 McLeod Cancer Report reflects 2014 cancer data at McLeod Regional Medical Center. This information includes the results of clinical quality efforts and outstanding progress by the physicians and nursing staff of the McLeod Oncology team. The report also provides specific data on lung cancer, one of our top five cancer tumor sites, and a summary of the 1,410 cases of cancer diagnosed and treated at McLeod in 2014.

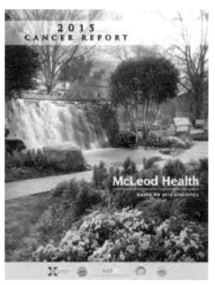

---

[4] For more information see: McLeod Cancer Resource Guide:
http://www.mcleodhealth.org/mrmc-florence/services-florence/cancer-report.html

Cancer Resource Guide[5]

The McLeod Cancer Resource Guide contains information about the medical staff, treatment options, technology, and programs and services that encompasses the McLeod Center for Cancer Treatment and Research. We hope you find this guide helpful and encouraging whether you are a patient, caregiver or physician.

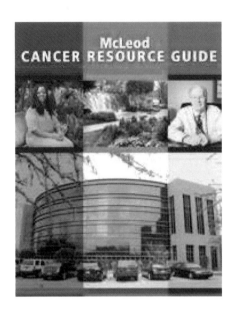

[5] For more information see: McLeod Cancer Resource Guide:
http://ddi7sqcxg475i.cloudfront.net/images/Mcleod_Florence/MRMC_PDFs/
McLeod%20Cancer%20Resource%20Guide.pdf

CHAPTER 8.   OVARIAN CANCER STAGES: WHAT ARE THE STAGES?[6]

Making an educated treatment decision begins with the stage, or progression, of the disease. The stage of ovarian cancer is one of the most important factors in evaluating treatment options.

Our cancer doctors use a variety of diagnostic tests to evaluate ovarian cancer and develop an individualized treatment plan. If you have been recently diagnosed, we will review your pathology to confirm you have received the correct diagnosis and staging information, and develop a personalized treatment plan. If you have a recurrence, we will perform comprehensive testing and identify a treatment approach that is suited to your needs.

TNM system for ovarian cancer
The ovarian cancer staging process uses the TNM system:

- **Tumor (T)** describes the size of the original tumor.
- **Lymph Node (N)** indicates whether the cancer is present in the lymph nodes.
- **Metastasis (M)** refers to whether cancer has spread to other parts of the body, usually the liver, bones or brain.

Once the T, N and M scores have been assigned, an overall ovarian cancer stage is assigned.

Stage I ovarian cancer
In stage I ovarian cancer, the cancer is limited to one or both ovaries. Stage I is broken into three separate subcategories:

- **IA**: Cancer is confined to one ovary. No cancer cells are present on the surface of the ovary or in the pelvis or abdomen.
- **IB**: Cancer is present inside both ovaries, but no cancer cells are present on the surface of the ovaries, in the pelvis or the abdomen.

---

[6] http://www.cancercenter.com/ovarian-cancer/stages/

- **IC**: Cancer is present in one or both of the ovaries. In addition, cancer cells are present on the surfaces of one or both ovaries, one tumor has ruptured or cancer cells are found in fluid samples from the abdomen.

Stage II ovarian cancer
Stage II ovarian cancer means that the disease has spread from the ovary to the pelvic organs, such as the fallopian tubes or uterus. Stage II has three subcategories:

- **IIA**: Cancer is present in one or both of the ovaries and has spread into the uterus or fallopian tubes. No cancer cells are present in the abdomen.
- **IIB**: Cancer is present in one or both of the ovaries and has spread to other pelvic organs, such as the bladder, colon or rectum.
- **IIC**: Cancer is present in one or both ovaries, and the cancer has spread to the pelvic organs and is found in fluid samples from the abdomen.

Stage III
In stage III, the cancer has spread from the ovary and beyond the pelvis to the abdomen or nearby lymph nodes. This stage has three subcategories:

- **IIIA**: Cancer is present in one or both of the ovaries, and cancer cells are also present in microscopic amounts in the abdominal fluid.
- **IIIB**: Cancer is present in one or both of the ovaries, and cancer cells are also present in tumors smaller than 2 cm in the abdominal lining.
- **IIIC**: Cancer is present in one or both of the ovaries, and cancer cells are also present in tumors larger than 2 cm in the abdominal lining or in the nearby lymph nodes.

Stage IV
Stage IV ovarian cancer means that the disease has spread from the ovary to distant sites in the body, such as the liver or lungs.

Recurrent ovarian cancer
Recurrent or relapsed ovarian cancer occurs when malignant cells reappear after cancer treatments such as surgery or chemotherapy have been completed for a

period of time. Recurrent ovarian cancer may return at its original location, or it may be found somewhere else in the body.

Ovarian cancer typically recurs when a small number of cancer cells survive the treatment process but are not detected on tests. After treatment, these cancer cells may grow into tumors. When ovarian cancer recurs in the ovaries, it is called a local recurrence. A regional relapse occurs when ovarian cancer cells are detected in the lymph nodes. When it develops in other parts of the body, such as the bone or brain, it is called a distant recurrence. Both regional relapse and distant recurrence are considered metastatic ovarian cancer.

The signs of recurrent ovarian cancer may vary from patient to patient. Because the ovaries are located near the bladder and the intestines, gastrointestinal symptoms typically develop.

Signs and symptoms of local ovarian cancer recurrence may include:

- Persistent abdominal bloating, indigestion or nausea
- Changes in appetite, typically a loss of appetite or feeling full sooner
- Pressure in the pelvis or lower back
- Urge to urinate more frequently
- Changes in bowel movements
- Increased abdominal girth

Signs and symptoms of metastatic ovarian cancer may include:

- Lethargy, fatigue or lack of energy
- Abdominal pain or swelling
- Swelling or lumps in the lymph nodes
- Unexplained pain in other areas of the body, such as the bones
- Elevated levels of the protein CA-125

According to the Ovarian Cancer National Alliance, an estimated 70 percent of patients diagnosed with ovarian cancer develop a recurrence. The cancer recurrence rate varies by patient, but the risk increases with the cancer's stage at the time it was originally diagnosed (the more advanced the stage, the higher the risk). Follow-up appointments with your oncologist may help detect cancer relapse early. Routine gynecologic care and annual pelvic exams are recommended to screen for symptoms of relapsed ovarian cancer.

CHAPTER 9.   INFORMING YOUR FAMILY & FRIENDS

Well, telling my family and friends about my health condition wasn't exactly what I had in mind. But I had to do it, some way, some how. Keeping in mind that this was devastating news and, being calm while informing them, was my main priority. No problem at all...

Husband:

My Sweetie was with me when we were given the news. You took the dreaded news of my illness like a champ and became my #1 supporter. Thanks honey.

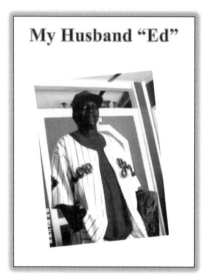

My Husband "Ed"

And here I thought I would've been taking care of my man when *he* got older. But think again. The world has changed and age ain't nothing but a number. I'm currently 55 and he's 74. Today, our loving and respectable relationship has lasted for 20 years. Ed, being 18-plus years my senior, is in better shape than any young stud I know. How does he care for me with so many things on his plate?

Massaging my body on a regular basis
Making sure I make my doctor appointments
Making sure I take my daily medication
Bathing/Dressing

Dusting
Sweeping
Mopping floors
Vacuuming
Washing dishes
Cooking/Preparing meals
Doing laundry
Cleaning bathrooms
Watering plants
Mowing the lawn
Taking out the trash
Washing the car
Clothes shopping
Food shopping
and etc.

Even though my husband was receiving retirement income, it was barely enough for us to get by on. My income was the sugar and cream to our coffee and when it ran out, the coffee was never the same. We were going through something awful and weird at the same time. Together as a team, we always brought home the bacon and fried it up in a pan. But now we had to figure out how to manage living off of one income while using the same old frying pan. Well, this too did pass. Thank you Lord for helping us to stay strong. *Amen.*

Today, my sweetie continues to care for me. It must be love. Remember, never underestimate the elderly. They are capable of handling their business when the need arises! Much love to you, honey. You are the best!

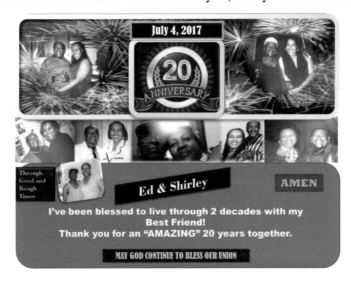

On our honeymoon week in the summer of 2010, we happily invited the family to join us in celebrating this very special event. And although we may have shared many laughs together, I think my sweetie had something else on his mind. LOL.

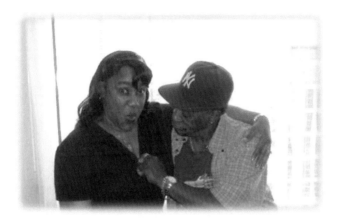

In late 2009, we decided to get creative and show each other how to have a little fun. We dressed up like a young, fun-loving couple and expressed our undying love for one another. *Amen.*

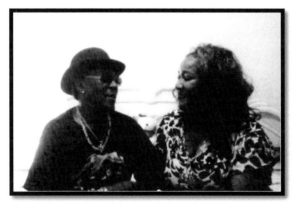

Just like his mother, Ed was born and raised in Virginia. Back in the '40s you didn't have today's choice of talking back to adults. Coming from a single parent household, lessons were learned at the early age of eight for my husband. In those times, he would have to look up to his mother when she called his name. His mother wore an apron tied tightly around her waist, and as she cooked, my husband would constantly tug on that apron, while, at the same time, inquire about the ingredients of the food she was preparing. She would then give him a little nudge, escort him aggressively into another room and have him read a book. Obviously, Ed had no other choice but to read because television wasn't an option at that time. LOL. According to my husband, his mother didn't allow disrespect either, especially from her children. Therefore, you did what you were told and that's just the way things were. *Amen.*

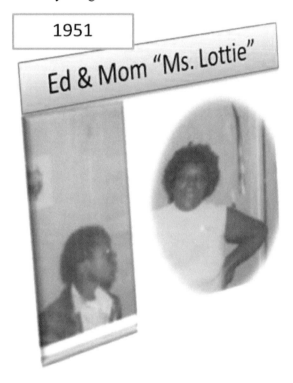

1951

Ed & Mom "Ms. Lottie"

I guess nagging your mom for a little affection while she's cooking, does pay off after all. And although Ed was raised in a fatherless home, he turned out to be an outstanding individual who knows the meaning of love and respect. I never had any idea at the start of our relationship that today, it would be stronger than it ever was before. He continues to treat me as a queen and his mom did a splendid job in raising him. At this point, the only statement I could make is: "His Momma sure raised him right!" Thank you Ms. Lottie for raising a well-respected young man. May you continue to rest in peace. *Amen.*

My Sisters:

Baby Sister Gail was the first on the scene once she received the news. With me living in South Carolina and her in Georgia, I heard she didn't hesitate to "floor it" when it was time to visit her ill sister in the hospital.

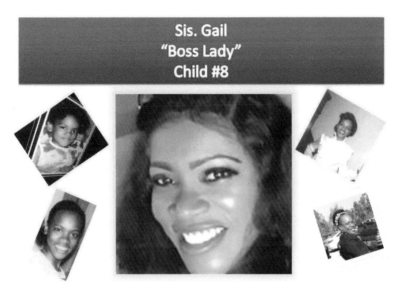

Sis. Gail
"Boss Lady"
Child #8

To Gail: On that day, you brought a gift basket full of surprises. I'll never forget what was inside. There were slippers, a toothbrush, toothpaste, lotion, a nightgown and other personal items. I appreciated them all. But the nightgown wasn't a regular nightgown, it was an *inspirational* nightgown. The gown was full-length, short-sleeved and green, with an engraved embossed writing saying "RELAX! *God's in Charge*" which I absolutely adored.

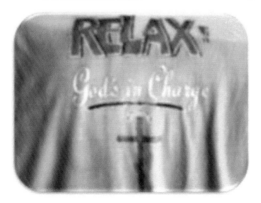

To this day, I continue to wear that nightgown. And yes, you were so right — God was (and is) in charge and there was absolutely nothing I could do about it, except follow my doctor's orders. But the best gift of all was your visit which comprised a great deal of laughs, cries, hugs and kisses along the way. I'd especially like to thank you for helping me with all the paperwork while I was hospitalized. Ha, ha. Love you Sis. Thanks for those beautiful and memorable moments. *Amen.*

It's sad but up until my sickness, my baby sister and I hadn't been close for some years now. As sisters we were always in competition with one another, and sometimes these things don't always turn out right. But at the end of the day, family will always be there for one another. And if I may say so myself, my sickness miraculously brought us back together — even closer than ever. It's really not important how the confusion in our relationship began, but what is important is that no matter the situation, we will love and be there for one another.

Not sure if I've ever told you, but I've always admired you for your spunk, wittiness and braveness for being one of the baddest women I know. You are a boss lady, running a family business while at the same time taking notes and kicking butts. My baby sister worked very hard to become the entrepreneur in our family. I will always love and respect you. *Amen.*

And, on this particular day, as a little girl, you kept the adults entertained because they were surely impressed with what you had to say. *Amen.*

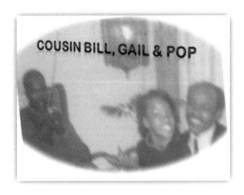

COUSIN BILL, GAIL & POP

Through God, you've blessed this family with two handsome and intelligent sons, Matthew the eldest, and Kevin Jr. the youngest.

Matthew
Grandchild #10

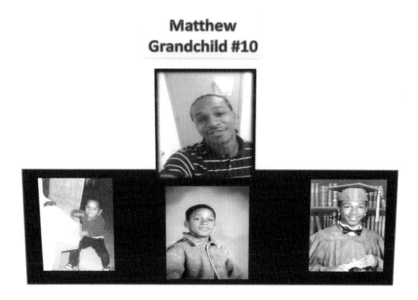

Matthew has continued the family legacy and has blessed our family with two adorable boys, Matthew Jr. and Makhi. Unfortunately, I haven't physically met my grandnephews but understand they both enjoy attending school and live very full and exciting lives. And, thanks to Facebook, I can actually see posts and hear videos of these precious little guys.

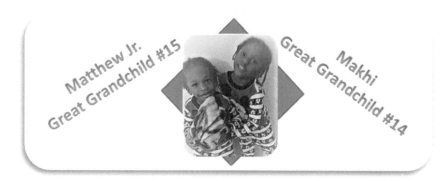

Matthew Jr.
Great Grandchild #15

Great Makhi
Grandchild #14

Matthew and his beautiful soulmate Yonnie, insist on showing their children how to take the right paths in life — whether by keeping in shape, or paying close attention to their schoolwork. Either way, they both have given their children a healthy and stable environment to grow up in. May you both continue to be blessed, and I pray that one day soon, I will have the opportunity to see this part of my family real soon. God bless. *Amen.*

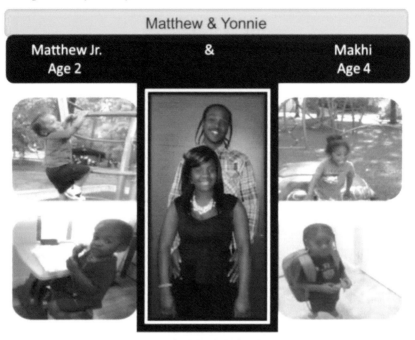

Kevin Jr.
Grandchild #11

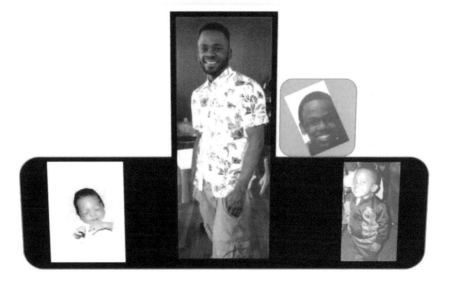

Middle Sister Linda showed me so much love and support.

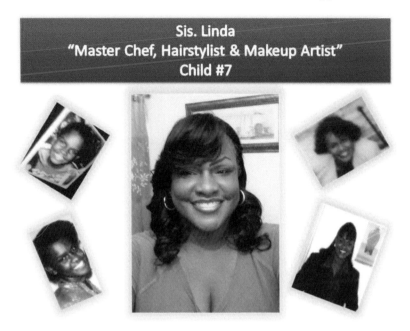

Sis. Linda
"Master Chef, Hairstylist & Makeup Artist"
Child #7

To Linda: While visiting, you cooked, cleaned, and accompanied me to doctor's visits while nurturing me back to good health with your great but crazy sense of humor. Love you Sis. Always.

As well, you also prepared attractive and delicious meals and we enjoyed them to the fullest. My husband and I appreciated it all. Thanks Sis.

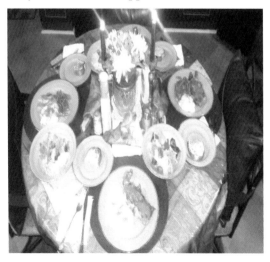

Growing up, Linda had always been known as the "hair queen" in our neighborhood. Back in the day, she would perform cornrows, weaves, extensions and other hairstyles for family, friends and individuals she didn't even know. She would also provide cornrows and haircuts to the neighborhood guys as well. Linda was also good in applying makeup. So, of course, with all of her experience, she played a very important role in my hair loss. After losing my hair, Linda would send me wigs, scarves, turbans and hats to lift up her big sister's spirits. Losing my hair did depress me but she would try anything to cheer me up. When visiting, she would apply makeup to my face and touch up my hair to make me feel better about myself. I will always be grateful to her.

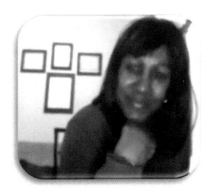

On my down days, Linda would always try to cheer me up. We would do things like play board games such as Bingo, checkers and Scrabble. When it came time for other games such as blackjack, poker, and slots, they were played on the Internet. We would also watch funny TV shows to keep both our spirits up. Other times we would go to Walmart to shop for food and other necessities.

Linda had me on the floor laughing one day when she came to visit. We had both decided to play the board game Bingo and I just so happened to win five games in a row. She actually got a little upset and started to pout — just like when we were little. I thought that was the cutest thing ever. And if anybody could take me back to sibling rivalry, it would be her, because that's what sisters do: stay on one's nerve while loving each other at the same time. Thanks for all of your support. Love you Sis. Always.

<u>Big Sister Renita</u> was the first to be told and she then informed the others.

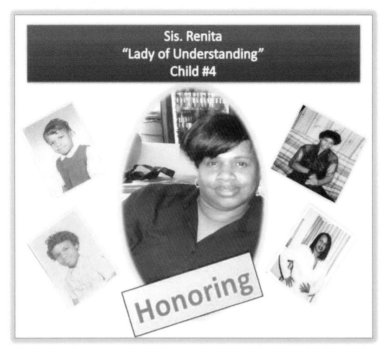

To Renita: You've always been the oldest and the shyest of us four girls. And although you weren't involved in Facebook at the time, you did manage to inform family and friends of my illness. And through the help from others on Facebook, additional family and friends were informed. Thanks for being a stand-up sister and passing the word to our loved ones.

When I informed you of my not feeling well prior to diagnosis, you made certain that I go directly to the hospital ASAP. How in the world did you know that would be the most important decision I'll ever make in my entire life? God bless you Sis.

I admire you for your bravery in helping me to fight this battle. Momma would be so proud of you today. You have taken on some of her wonderful and motherly qualities in caring for others. When I needed to talk — you were always there to listen. When I needed a shoulder to cry on — you were always there for me. When I needed to pray — you always prayed with me.

Today and always, I am honoring you, for being there for me through the most vulnerable time of my life. I couldn't have held it down without your understanding of my illness and the situation surrounding it. Thank you for being a special kind of sister. All of my years on this planet, you have shown me nothing but love, loyalty and dedication as a big sister. Thank you for being a special kind of sister. Love always Sis. *Amen.*

I'm also honoring you for your love, loyalty and dedication that you give wholeheartedly and unconditionally to your grandchildren. They have been blessed to have a wonderful grandmother in their lives.

You also have helped to create one fabulous daughter who has achieved so much love in her life. Even as a little girl, Michelle had a great deal of potential and showed early signs of maturity. Although she was more mature than others in her age group, she had a loveable and fun sense of humor. Her

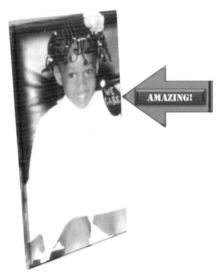

beauty and smile would capture your attention every time she'd walk into a room. She would slowly and meticulously keep her eyes and ears open for anything exciting and new. This little girl paid attention in life and the signs began at an early age. Today, the same methods apply — caring for others. Just see the "WE CARE" sticker pinned to the top left side of her dress. Amazing!

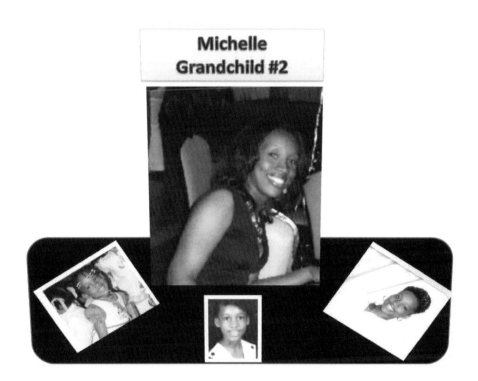

Michelle
Grandchild #2

I've always considered William and Michelle as the power couple of the decade. You two got together, made plans and goals and worked very diligently on achieving them. When something in life threw you a curve ball, you two found a way to catch it! That's my beautiful family. Wow!

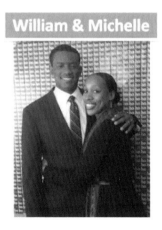

William & Michelle

Through their loving support, I have recognized not only my needs, but the needs of others. William and Michelle are raising two wonderful children.

While Shayla is currently attending middle school with honors, she is also bright, beautiful and a mirror image of her mother.

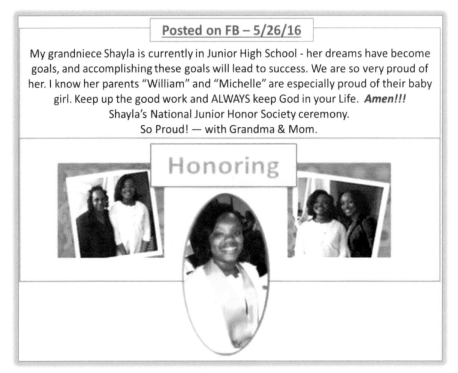

Posted on FB – 5/26/16

My grandniece Shayla is currently in Junior High School - her dreams have become goals, and accomplishing these goals will lead to success. We are so very proud of her. I know her parents "William" and "Michelle" are especially proud of their baby girl. Keep up the good work and ALWAYS keep God in your Life. *Amen!!!* Shayla's National Junior Honor Society ceremony. So Proud! — with Grandma & Mom.

Even during the family's personal religious time, William is persistent in watching over his children carefully, guiding Shayla in the right direction. God is always on time when you focus on what really matters in life. *Amen.*

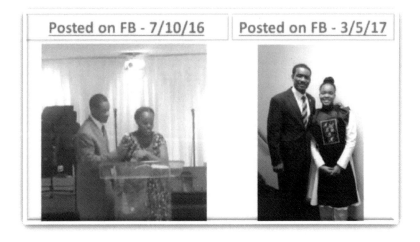

Posted on FB - 7/10/16   Posted on FB - 3/5/17

This is what family time is all about — spending precious time together while praising His name. *Amen.*

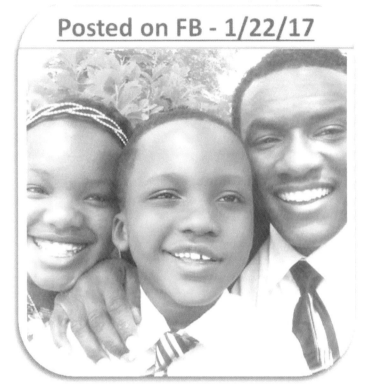

Posted on FB - 1/22/17

Their son William Jr. was diagnosed with autism at an early age. He is currently 11 years of age and is very close to his older sister Shayla. William and Michelle are dedicated in providing William Jr. with the necessary services for his improvement. In addition, love, attention and prayer are their main priorities. William and Michelle are strong individuals who believe in never giving up on their family.

William Jr. is very active in his everyday life but must be supervised at all times. He is, however, a lot smarter than people think. William Jr. is adorable, loving, funny and at times, a little rough and other times, a little soft. But with patience, understanding, love and prayers, our family will be all right. Remember: There is so much to learn about autism and much knowledge we can share with others. *Amen.*

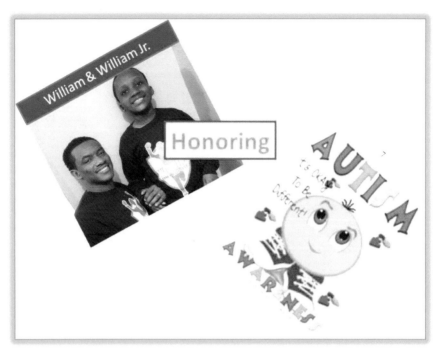

8

What is Autism ?

Autism is a lifelong developmental disability that affects how a person communicates with, and relates to, other people. It also affects how they make sense of the world around them.

It is a spectrum condition, which means that, while all people with autism share certain difficulties, their condition will affect them in different ways.

Tagged/Created by
Kimberly Photo K

---

[7] https://www.pinterest.com/pin/526358275170418817/
[8] https://www.pinterest.com/claudiastanley/autism-awareness/

Always

Unique

Totally

INtEREStiNG

Sometimes

Mysterious

Again, like always, William shows love and support to his children. William Jr. continues to accelerate in learning the skills and safety of swimming. He is assisted with help while at the same time, making progress. God bless you grand-nephew. Your family is highly impressed with the improvement in your achievements. *Amen.*

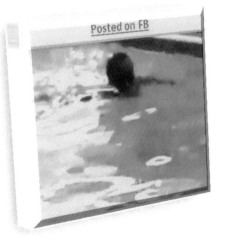

Posted on FB

---

[9] http://thisability.org/yahoo_site_admin/assets/images/37328_autism.253152353_std.jpg

Shayla
Great Grandchild #7

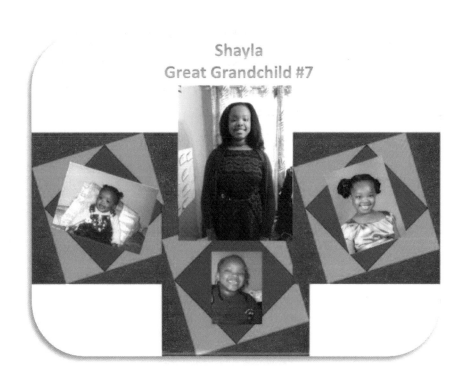

William Jr.
Great Grandchild #9

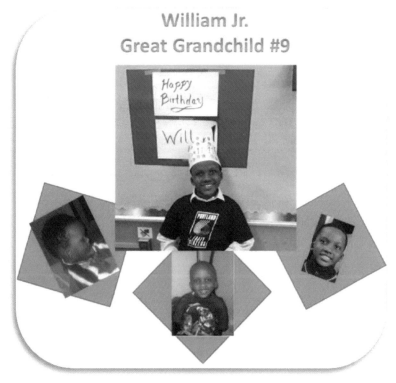

This beautiful family devotes quality time together, especially during the holiday season. It's a miracle to experience the pleasure of watching my family share happy memorable moments together. Thank God we believe in putting family first. *Amen.*

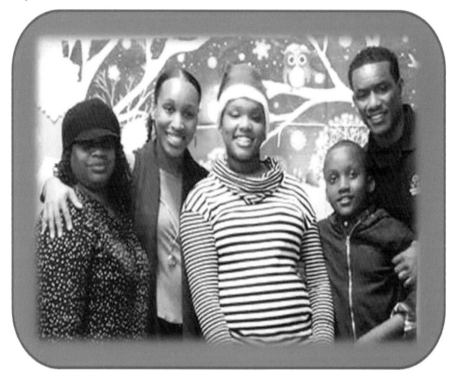

The feeling of being able to return the love and support is overwhelming. I get so excited and deeply emotional every time I notice a photo or video on Facebook of my family — attending events and achieving their goals. Actually seeing Shayla and William Jr. grow and mature online, is amazing! Picking up the phone or doing a Facebook video chat always seem to be our answer to sharing family moments.

Thank you creator of Facebook for creating such a website that helps to bring our family closer together, even when we're physically apart. God bless Michelle and William, for they are a blessing to our family. *Amen.*

When my sisters came to visit in August 2015, it was happily more than I could stand. What a blast we had sharing hugs and kisses, happiness and good eating. And just think of all the fun we had! Getting love and support from my lovely sisters.

Back in the day, when we were growing up, it was all about dolls, hopscotch and jacks. Today, it's all about enjoying yourself on your computer, laptop or even a cell phone. My sisters and I played fun games with one another in my game room. We were like kids all over again.

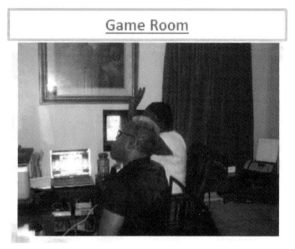

Doing our usual thing and posing for Jet Magazine. Ha, ha, ha.

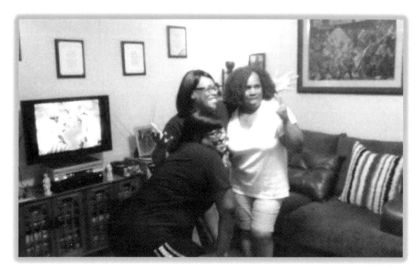

Big sister Renita would sometimes use her cell phone to play fun games.

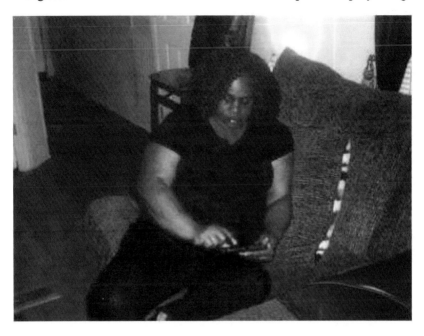

I've always enjoyed visits from my sisters. It's the goodbyes that get to me the most.

Me & Sis. Gail

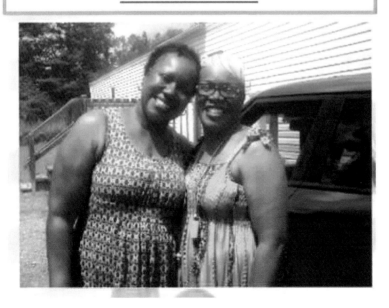

My sister Linda insisted on keeping a smile on my face during this sad time. I know I'm not the easiest person to get along with but you gave me all the love and support I needed.

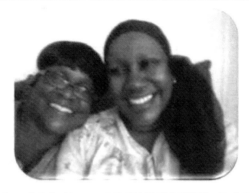

Sis. Linda & Me

Thanks for the visit ladies — THIS IS HOW WE DO IT!

Again, in September 2016, my baby sister Gail came to visit. We had such a wonderful time, we couldn't control ourselves. You know we had to post it all on Facebook. How else were we supposed to show our support for one another? If anybody could make me smile and laugh like a clown, it would be my baby sister Gail. Thanks for everything girl — I love you to the fullest! God bless you.

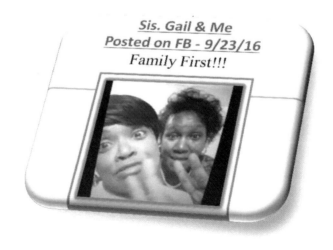

Sis. Gail & Me
Posted on FB - 9/23/16
Family First!!!

Just having a blessed weekend with my baby sister on Facebook. We were enjoying the beautiful weather as well as each other's company. Concentrating on love, life and laughter, as we say our goodbyes on this visit.

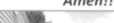

Sis. Gail & Me
Posted on FB - 9/25/16
BLESSED WEEKEND – I'm so glad we had this time together,
just to have a laugh, or sing a song.
Seems we just get started and before you know it,
comes the time we have to say, "So long".
Until Next Time Little Sister – May God Always Be With You...
Amen!!!

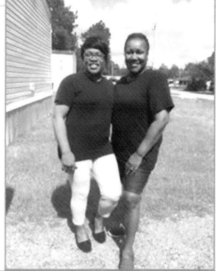

Things have changed a great deal today with everyone living in different states and all. But I'll have to admit, with the progress in technology and with Skype and social media such as Facebook, Twitter, Instagram and others, folks have no excuse for not staying in touch with their loved ones. *Amen.*

So ladies, no matter where we are in life or death, the awesome foursome sisters remain unstoppable! *Amen.*

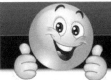 # Me & My Sisters

Over 50

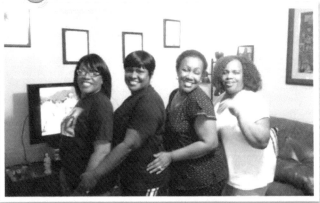

Late 30s to Mid 40s

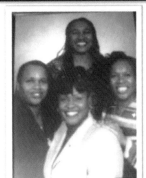

Early to Late 30s

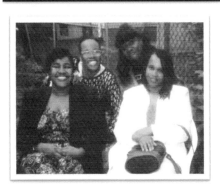

Late Teens to Early 20s

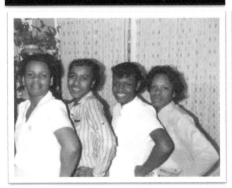

Early to Late Teens

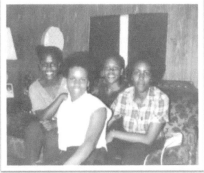

Son NahDreams:

How do you tell your one and only son that you've been diagnosed with ovarian cancer? I only vaguely recall the exact words used, but I do remember his response and his facial expression. In all the years he's been on this earth, this is the first time I've ever seen NahDreams look as if he had lost his closest friend. And I see why — I was his closest friend. The love and bond between a mother and son is forever precious and should never be broken. I believe NahDreams was scared and afraid of losing me and afraid of the pain and suffering I would have to endure. Being mindful of my situation — what a blessing he is.

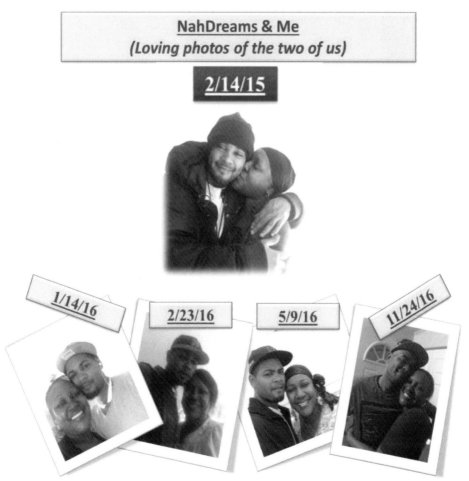

NahDreams & Me
(Loving photos of the two of us)

2/14/15

1/14/16   2/23/16   5/9/16   11/24/16

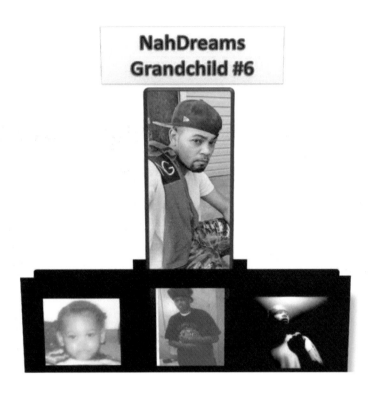

NahDreams
Grandchild #6

As a teenager, you and I experienced our first Caribbean Cruise together. I thought I'd never be taking that ride. For as long as I can remember, I have always shied away from cruises. My preference for being on land as opposed to water was always more comforting. The thought of riding on boats, ships and yachts always seem to make me feel queasy. Sad, but I think the fear of drowning has prevented me from taking these types of trips. But, there are some things in life you just have to try once, and so we did.

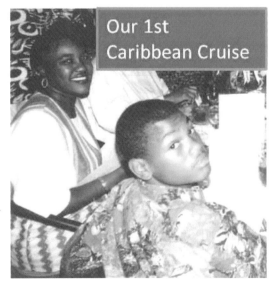

Our 1st Caribbean Cruise

I want to thank you Lord for blessing me and my family with a loving and safe trip to the Caribbean. We had a beautiful time and will never forget the happiness we shared. *Amen.*

Even as a little guy you were right there by my side:

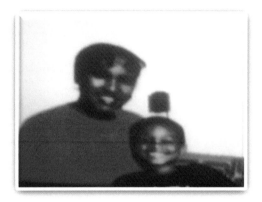

And as a toddler, you were more than a handful to manage. But you always kept a smile.

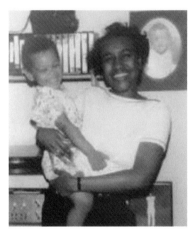

To NahDreams: Thanks for all your love and support. You have been there for me through thick and thin. You will forever be in my heart. *God bless.*

NahDreams has always been a loving and caring son. My knight in shining armor. My protector. All through your years you've resembled your father, but today I can fairly say that you are his clone. You were 13 when he passed away and now you are about the same age he was when he departed this life. And even though we can't physically hear or touch him, he will always be remembered in our hearts.

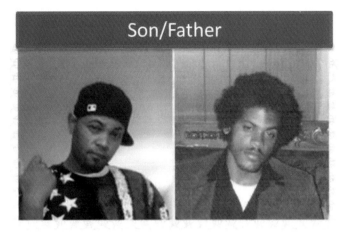
Son/Father

Willie Jr. (a/k/a Big Naheen or Junior) and I both met and resided in Jamaica, Queens. At that time, I was attending my last year of high school while he worked at the neighborhood gas station. And on my way to school I had to walk past the same gas station in order to catch the school bus. My goal was to always get to school on time. But everyday, I would walk by this gas station and Big Naheen would insist on talking to me. Even while pumping customer's gas, he would talk to me. I couldn't believe the nerve 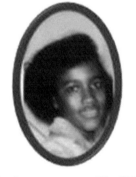 of this guy and I would totally ignore him. I was young and naïve and I wasn't interested in anyone at that time. However, he would continuously bother me every day, Monday through Friday, while asking the silliest questions. Things like: "What's your name?"; "Can you stop walking away while I'm talking to you?"; "Can we get together?"; "Why are you ignoring me?"; and so on. Then, eventually, he finally got my attention by saying: "Hey girl, it's my birthday today. Can I get a kiss on the cheek?" Yeah, I went for it all right. But when I reached to give him that kiss, he quickly turned his head so that both of our lips would meet. The only way I could respond was to laugh,

83

walk away and eventually date the little rascal. By the way, it wasn't even his birthday that day. Ha, ha, ha.

Later, that following December, we found out I was pregnant. And when we informed our family, my Pop decided that we were going to have a shotgun wedding.

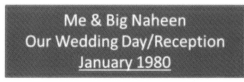

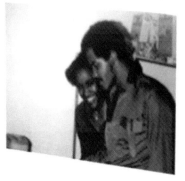

Me & Big Naheen
Our Wedding Day/Reception
January 1980

And seven months later, after our wedding, NahDreams was born. We were so very proud to bring another human being into this world; to love and care for someone we needed and who needed us.

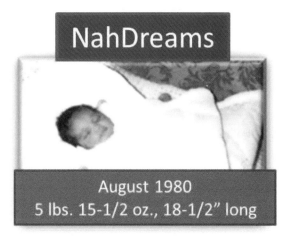

NahDreams

August 1980
5 lbs. 15-1/2 oz., 18-1/2" long

AND THE REST IS HISTORY!

My Brothers:

Oldest Brother Terry found out about my illness through our Brother Jeffrey, and he found out through our sisters. It was 2015, but quite special to have both my brothers call me to check on the status of my health. I enjoyed our conversation so much that it actually made me cry because I haven't seen or heard from these two for quite some time.

To Terry and Jeffrey: I know your lives are currently hectic and complicated, but I've been praying to God to provide good health and happiness to both of you. I miss you both and hope and pray that you are doing well. May God bless you and keep you safe. *Amen.*

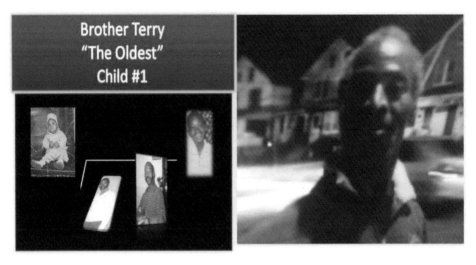

Although Jeffrey has been staying in touch with me over the years, it's been a few months since I last heard from him. But thanks to Facebook, I was able to see and speak with him via Facebook video chat. We had such a wonderful and talkative time, laughing and joking about the good times and how anxious we were while planning our next visit with one another. Going forward, Jeffrey and I will be following Facebook as a tool for communication. The importance of keeping and staying in touch in our family means a lot to us. Thank you God for giving us this beautiful blessing to share together. *Amen.*

Posted on FB - 2/15/17

In addition to waking up bright and early this morning by the grace of God, I was so delighted to have received a video call from my brother Jeffrey who I haven't seen for some years now. I have to thank Facebook for providing a way for folks to reach out to their loved ones. *Amen.*

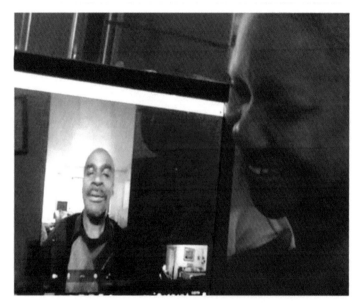

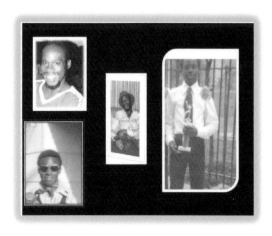

Growing up as kids, Jeffrey was my protector. He's one year older and we attended the same schools and shared the same friends. Sometimes, when I was being teased by classmates, Jeffrey would confront them nicely and asked that they not do such a thing. I was glad to have an older brother to look after me while growing up.

During our elementary school days we were involved in many sports including gymnastics, handball and basketball, and Jeffrey would come home with trophies for winning tournaments.

Thank you for blessing this family with Momma and Pop's third born grandchild. And although you haven't heard from your son in a while, I fortunately did. Through Facebook, he was able to contact me through video chat and what a blessing it was to hear from him. We had a healthy and respectable conversation, and going forward, he will try to stay more in touch with the family. *Amen.*

Tony
Grandchild #3

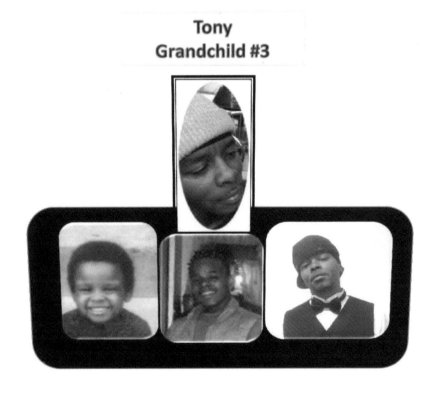

Brother David: It was the early afternoon of July 24, 1989, and baby sister Gail's 25th birthday. I was 27 at the time and David was 34. Gail and I planned to take off from work that day to celebrate her birthday, until the phone rang. It was Momma and she forgot to record her soap operas prior to leaving for work that day. Momma's VCR wasn't working at that time, so she instructed me to record it on David's device. David resided in the basement of Momma's house and should have already left for work. So, I agreed to tape Momma's soap operas and proceeded downstairs to the basement. When I arrived at the bottom of the stairs, I noticed the ceiling lights were still on. I said to myself: "This isn't right! David never, ever leaves his lights

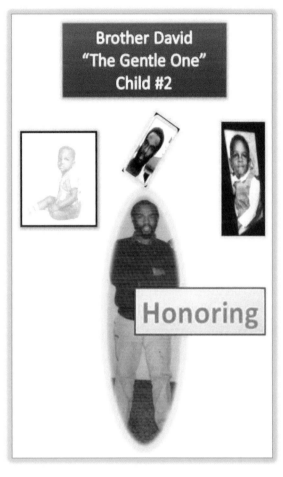

on when he goes to work. Maybe he just forgot to turn them off." But as I continued to walk toward the back of the basement which led to the bathroom, it appeared that the door was ajar, and near the entrance doorway lay a partial foot.

OMG! "It's David! He must have had a seizure!" I said aloud. He was lying on the bathroom floor, somewhat dressed in his work uniform. I went over to his body, and as I motioned to touch him, there was an aura of calmness, but yet a light coolness in the air. And when I actually touched him, he was cold as ice, stiff and unresponsive. I knew deep down in my heart, this was more than one of his usual seizures. This was something altogether different. He was too cold to be alive.

Going through this unfortunate experience has altered our family forever. Sorrowful moments of our family will never be forgotten on this sad and tragic day. This was my second brother who was gone and I was the one who actually discovered him. Ironically, David was the second born out of eight children, and the second born to die. It wasn't the seizure per se that actually killed him — it was a broken neck. From what I understood, David didn't have the appropriate room to spasm during the seizure. Therefore, his neck broke while convulsing, and that was the cause of death. OMG! This was the death of my brother, and he was no longer with us. For him, it's been over twenty years of suffering with seizures, but now, the suffering has finally come to an end. David was now with God. *Amen.*

David was a strong individual who never gave up on getting through each day. It was told to me that he began having seizures in his early teens, subsequent to getting hit in the head with a baseball. From that moment on, he was unfortunately diagnosed with epilepsy which caused seizures. It was very difficult for him to live a normal life because you never knew when the seizures would appear. But that didn't stop him from living or having fun. When he attended junior high and high school he went through hell because of this illness. Constantly, the schools had to call Momma to report David's situation and eventually, he got fed up and discouraged and dropped out altogether. Shortly after, he did land a full-time position in Manhattan while working with a good friend. This friend gave good references and David was eventually employed. His employer never complained of his constant absences. They were aware of his illness prior to his hire and they understood the circumstances surrounding it. David was a good and dedicated worker and always took pride in getting up every morning to go to work. Prior to this death, he was employed for many years while working at the same company and was only absent on the days of his illness. *Amen.*

David was very active and enjoyed playing sports, and one of his favorites was basketball. Sometimes David would enter basketball tournaments and come home with trophies and awards for participating. At times, he would even actually win first prize trophies.

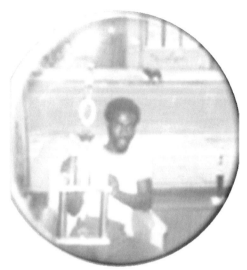

David loved to watch NBA and NFL sports on TV. His favorite TV comedy show was *Sanford and Son* because Redd Foxx was his idol. Despite every seizure he overcame, it was another day of enjoyment to treasure with his family. *Amen.*

On many occasions as an adult, David would begin his day by going to work, and ending it by being hospitalized. There were times Momma had to go to visit him in the hospital because of the seizures, especially the results of being found unconscious at subway stations, bus stops and other public places. One incident, I accompanied Momma in visiting David at the hospital. David demanded that Momma stop crying because this was the way it was. He would reiterate to Momma that he didn't have a life expectancy — only God knew when that would be. And how she and the family needed to stop worrying, and to be more prepared for when that time do come. We would brush it off and worry anyway, because that's what family does. We just didn't have any indication that this would be David's last and final seizure. It's always sad to lose a loved one, but when God prepares us, we should take notice and follow His lead. *Amen.*

There was one remarkable place David loved to attend on Sundays, and that was church. He would give glory to God every time he attended. Actually, it was my brother David who began attending and eventually joined our neighborhood church. As time went by, our entire family began joining the church. And just think, both LaSheena and NahDreams eventually attended the children's choir. First cousins, at early ages, were giving praises to our Lord. That was something special. *Amen.*

When David passed away, the church we all joined as a family presented both him and his daughter LaSheena with beautiful plaques in honor of their devotion and dedication to the church.

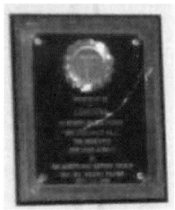

Today and always, I am honoring you, my brother David for your positive attitude and gentle approach on life, as you went through your constant struggle with epileptic seizures. First: for the support and protection you gave in raising a beautiful daughter (thank you God for not allowing David's illness to hinder the growth of our family); second: for bringing the family together as one in joining our community church; and third: for showing folks that just because you have an illness, it doesn't mean you can't live a fulfilling life.

Growing up, LaSheena was a beautiful and happy little lady. She was also the seventh grandchild born to Momma and Pop.

LaSheena
Grandchild #7

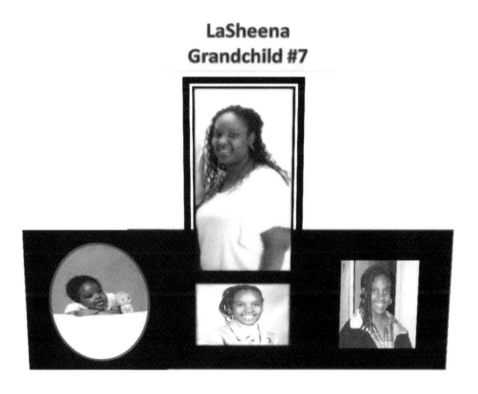

Today, your daughter LaSheena is all grown up and living the life. She and her husband Steve have created the "double trouble" team. If you team up on them, they will give you double the trouble. LOL. Not only do they protect one another, but they are protective of their parents as well. You would be so proud. Your grandchildren are adorable twin boys with smiles that can melt your heart away. I know

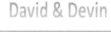

David & Devin

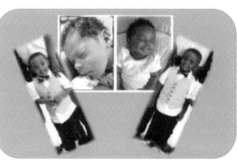

you are watching from up above because you helped to create a magnificent family. *Amen.*

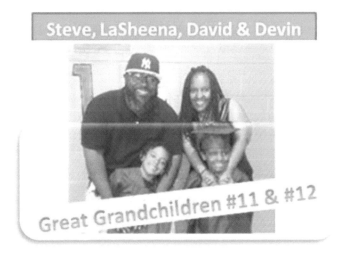

Steve, LaSheena, David & Devin

Great Grandchildren #11 & #12

Brother Steven: You were always known as "The Tough One." You refused to take any nonsense from any and everybody. You were in your early 20s when you left us and we've been missing you since. You and sister-in-law Evelyn have created Pop and Momma's dream of leaving a family legacy to carry on into the next generation. Give my sister-in-law a big shout-out for me and continue to rest in peace my brother, and your children will do the rest. *Amen.*

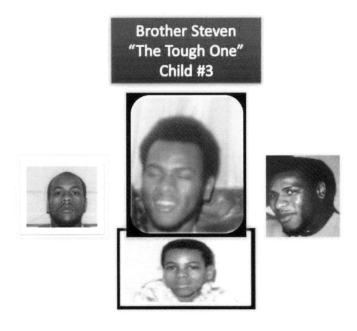

Brother Steven
"The Tough One"
Child #3

Sister-in-law Evelyn:

During my childhood years, my older brother Steven informed me of a new girlfriend. He said she had a beautiful smile and a head full of hair. He promised her that I would cornrow her hair because I was so good at braiding. So I agreed and we scheduled a date.

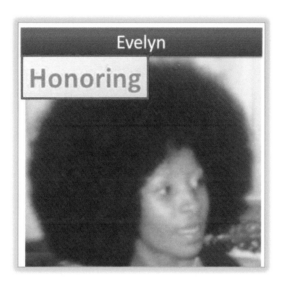

And there she was, Ms. Evelyn — young, gorgeous and with a head full of hair, just like my brother said. I took one look at her and said "no way was I braiding all that." I couldn't believe the amount of hair on her head. Her head resembled a forest overcrowded with trees, and, up until that point, I never had the opportunity to braid so much hair. But eventually I did. And what an honor it was! When I completed working on her hair, she was a queen in her own right. Beautiful as ever!

About one year later, I wanted my ears pierced just like the other girls in school. But Momma wasn't having it — she actually didn't wanna hear anything about it. But when Evelyn heard of my wishes, she volunteered to do the job herself. Eventually, Momma agreed and there I was, pierced and all. You have to remember, in those days all you needed was a needle, thread, peroxide and a little vaseline to create a masterpiece. I was so proud to be a girl who wore

94

earrings. It made me feel like a grown up and over the years, Evelyn and I shared great times together.

Evelyn was a beautiful and strong individual who loved Steven as well as their very first born. At times, Evelyn would slowly stare at Steven, gaze into his eyes and just love him unconditionally. With all that being said, I truly believe that my niece Leslie felt a little something-something too. LOL.

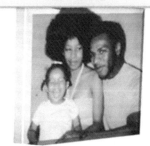

Evelyn, Steven & Leslie

Sadly, when my brother Steven departed this life, Evelyn was left to raise her three children alone. Although I was only eighteen at the time, I understood the sorrow my sister-in-law may have felt. Evelyn was three years my senior, but at times, would confide in me and my sisters. Evelyn would mention how lost and heartbroken she felt from the loss of my brother and how the meaning of their family unit was now gone. Evelyn was scared, afraid of trusting again, and confused about how to raise three children all on her own. At the end of the day, she was a young and struggling mother, just trying to make ends meet. But my family and I would assure her that we were behind her all the way.

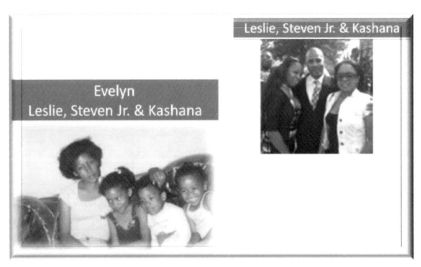

Evelyn
Leslie, Steven Jr. & Kashana

Leslie, Steven Jr. & Kashana

I remember on several occasions, my sisters and I would stop by Evelyn's home after school or work. Their home was located on the main drag and was easy to get there. We would spend quality time with our adorable nieces and nephew. Sometimes we would take them with us to the neighborhood donut shop where their father used to work.

Actually, the kids were young then, and when Steven passed away, Steven Jr. was only four months old. Kashana was about fifteen months old, and Leslie was five years old, and was responsible for helping to take care of her younger siblings. We love them all and frequently share family memories with them. Other favorite places to go when we would pick them up were the neighborhood pizza shop, the general store, and the hot dog vendor who was always standing on the corner of their home.

On many family occasions, great moments were spent with Evelyn and the kids. In this photo, Evelyn was more than delighted to share jokes and laughs with her sister-in-law Linda, and daughters Leslie and Kashana. We always treasured fond memories spent at Momma's house.

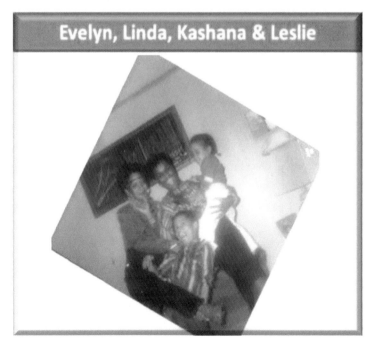

Evelyn, Linda, Kashana & Leslie

96

As time went by, Evelyn continued to raise her family to the best of her ability, and over the years, gave birth to two loving sons, John and Luis. They are the eighth and ninth grandchildren born to Momma and Pop. And, this was the beginning of *The Fabulous Five*.

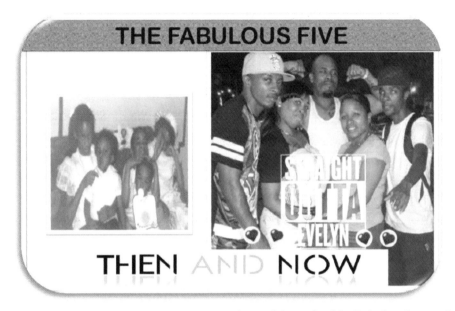

Even as a youngster, Steven Jr. showed love for his little brothers John and Luis. Steven Jr. would spend quality time with his brothers by taking them on bus trips to see other family members or just sharing good times together as a family.

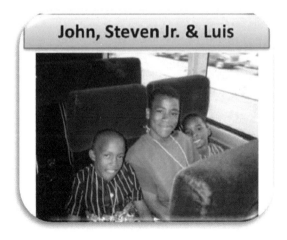

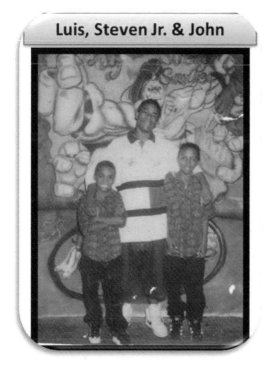

Luis, Steven Jr. & John

In 1986, Evelyn was diagnosed with breast cancer at the tender age of 28. During this time, Leslie was only eleven years of age and took on great responsibilities in helping to raise her siblings. Not only was Evelyn going through such a dramatic experience, so were her children. Uncertain whether their mom was going to pull through her illness, had to be very frightening for them especially at their young and tender ages. I can definitely relate to that entire situation completely.

However, over the years, Leslie has done a tremendous and outstanding job in helping to raise her siblings. To become an adult at an early stage in her life, due to illness in the family, had to be devastating for her. I can only imagine her confusion. But she did very well and has also, along with her siblings, display abundance of strength and unity toward family value because of it.

John and Luis are both adults now and have always been a part of our expanding family. Thank God we all had the pleasure of sharing fond memories together, and with many more to come. *Amen.*

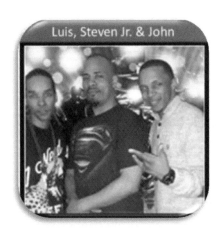

Luis, Steven Jr. & John

Evelyn fought this horrific battle for 24 years while going in and out of remission. So sad to say, she passed away in 2010 at the young age of 52. I know her battle was the most difficult and challenging experience she had to endure, but I'm so glad we as a family, were able to love her through it all. *Amen.*

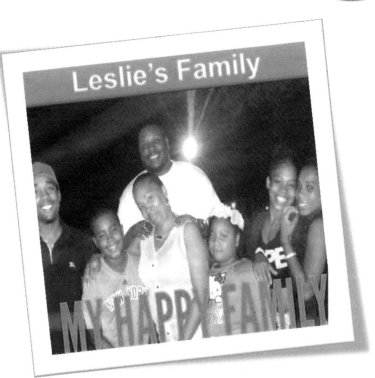

Leslie's Family

MY HAPPY FAMILY

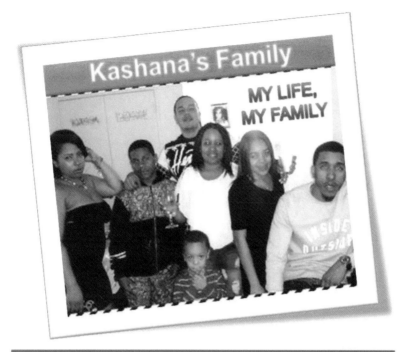

Kashana's Family

MY LIFE, MY FAMILY

Momma & Pop's
Grandchildren, Great Grandchildren
& Great Great-Grandchildren

Evelyn & Steven's
Children, Grandchildren and Great Grandchildren

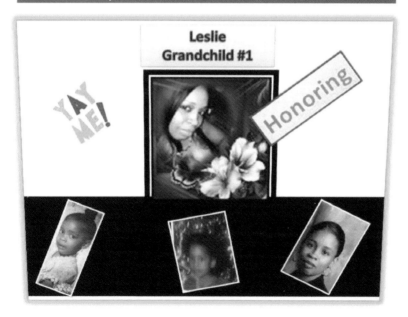

Leslie
Grandchild #1

YAY ME!

Honoring

To Leslie: I am honoring you for your strength in keeping the family together, especially after the loss of both your parents as well as the illness of your mother. Thanks for being strong and staying strong as like your grandma. This is what keeps our family more close than ever. *Amen.*

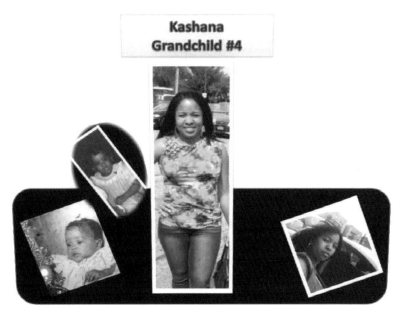

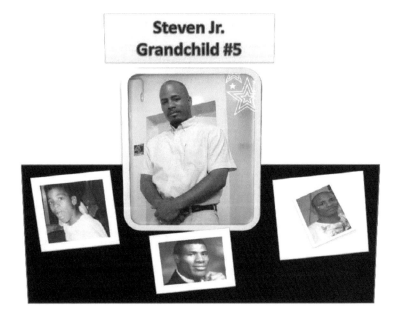

John
Grandchild #8

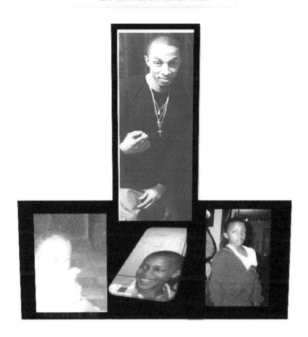

Luis
Grandchild #9

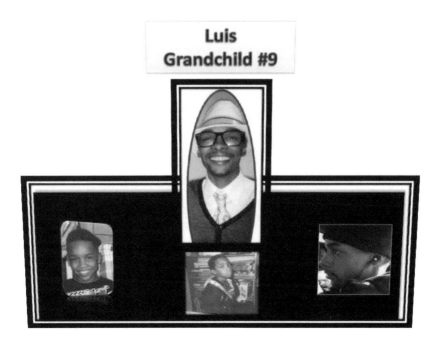

You and my brother Steven have been gone for quite some time now. But as time went by and your children became adults, the birth of a new generation began to emerge,

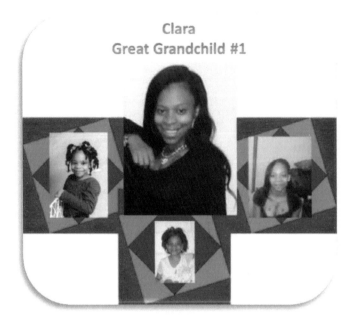

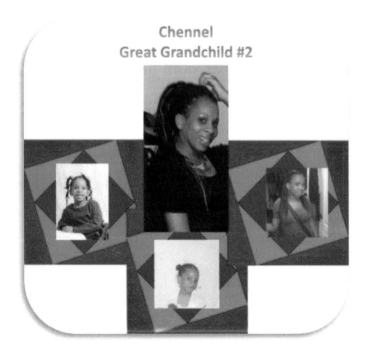

and then, another... That's right! Today, Evelyn and Steven would be great grandparents at early ages: Evelyn would be 58 and Steven 60 years of age. OMG!

These four little sweethearts are actually Pop & Momma's great great-grandchildren. OMG! Leslie's two daughters, Clara and Chennel, have created the next generation of our family legacy. This photo says to me: "Get ready 'cause here we come, and we come in *PEACE*!" LOL. May God bless my family (Emmanuel, Paradise, Zahir and Zamir). *Amen.*

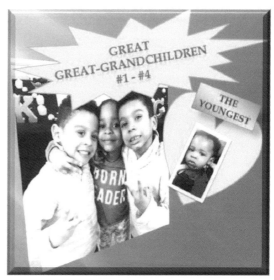

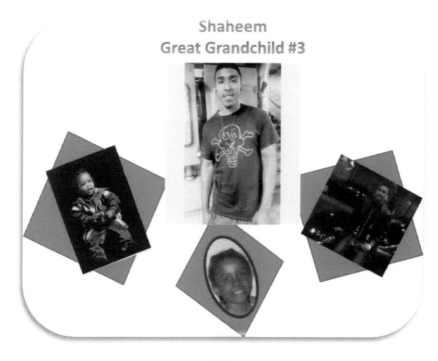

Shaheem
Great Grandchild #3

Naheem
Great Grandchild #4

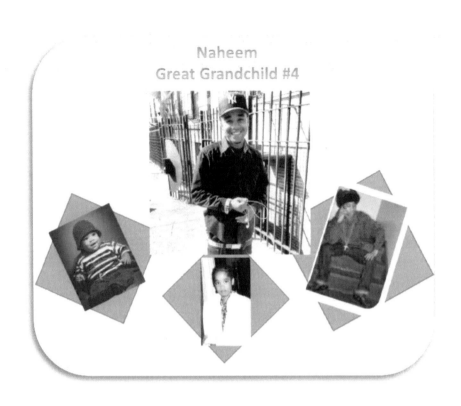

Evelyn
Great Grandchild #5

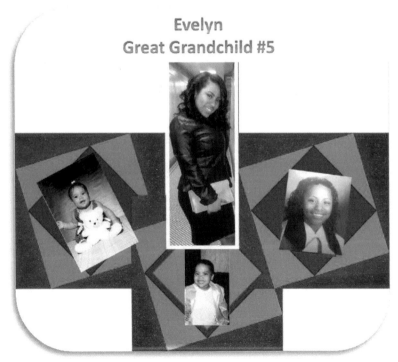

Selena
Great Grandchild #6

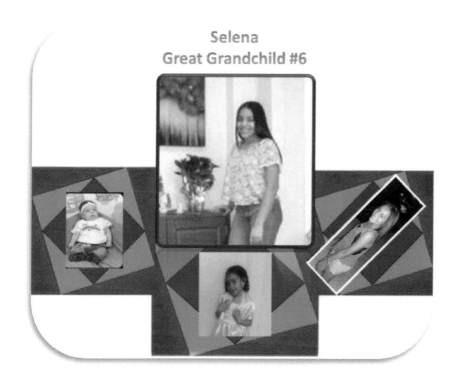

However, your granddaughter Selena has made family history. She manages to maintain excellent school grades, while at the same time, enter

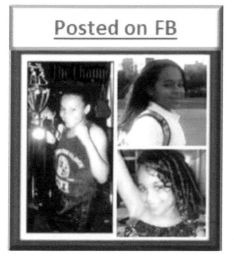

boxing tournaments as well as other events. She is also determined to become the very best at what she accomplishes. Her skills are magnificent and she carries a boxing style just like her grandpa Steven. Selena has also grown up to become a very beautiful and bright young lady just like her grandma Evelyn. Her determination in continuing to set and accomplish goals for herself is unbelievable at her young age. We, the family are very proud of you, and I know your grandparents are proud of you as well. Continue to be the sweet and studious lady that you are and always stay blessed. *Amen.*

Ni'zay
Great Grandchild #8

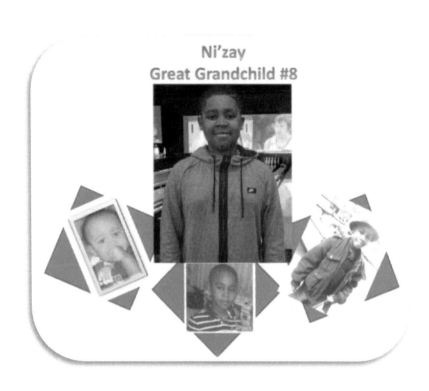

Ruby
Great Grandchild #10

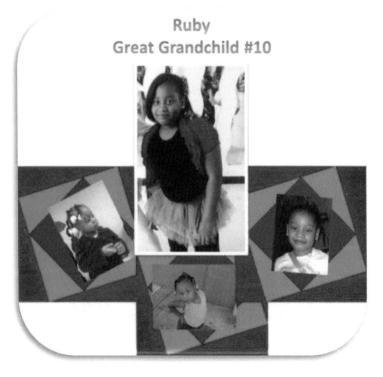

Leslie's daughter Ruby and son Ni'zay were little at this time, but until today, they continue to show love for one another. They look like little adults who have definitely been here before. God bless my grandniece and grandnephew. *Amen.*

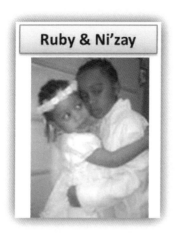

Little Ricky is having the time of his life as he enjoys taking his 5th birthday party photo shoot. He sure looked handsome and debonair, as he sports his dark jeans, white shirt and a bright blue bow tie. My grandnephew is a true model in the making, blowing up the screen with his intense, yet self-confident smile. The final touch was the hat, which was slightly slanted in a downward motion, on the right side, from the top to the bottom of his head. This little guy is going places and no

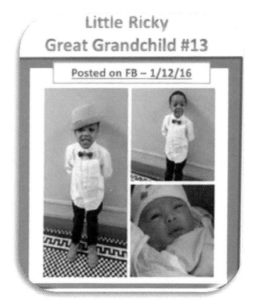

matter where, he'll be keeping the Lord with him. God bless my family for all the love given as well as received. *Amen.*

When Evelyn's brother passed away, and she lovingly helped to continue raising his son Elijah, the

family was honored. But then, when Evelyn passed, we were all at a loss and didn't know really where to turn. However, the family did come together to help raise Elijah, and eventually, his aunt Kashana became his legal guardian. Praise God! Kashana is a blessing because she is following her mother's dream in putting "Family First." It's exciting to know that Elijah is currently doing very well in school as well as sports. He strives in putting all of his energy, strength and training skills into his boxing goals. Continue to stay on top of the game Elijah. We love you dearly. God bless.

Leslie and Kashana continue to love and support one another as they share a special family moment with their loved ones, Tyrone and Rick. My nieces are in loving relationships with their soulmates, and today, have lasted for over seventeen years. God bless my family. *Amen.*

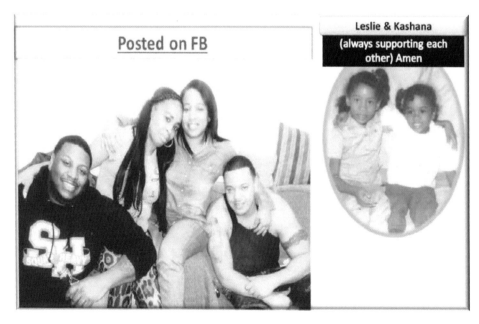

Leslie & Kashana
(always supporting each other) Amen

Steven Jr. and his soulmate Linda are in love as well, and have been for almost ten years, as they share their love with others on Facebook. *Amen.*

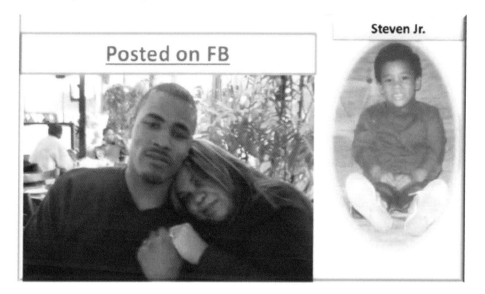

Thank you Evelyn for being the sister-in-law everyone wished they had. You fought your battle of breast cancer and you fought your battle of raising your children without a father. But God needed you more. You will always be blessed from above. *Amen.*

Girlfriend Sherrell:

Back in the '80s, I was working as a word processing supervisor for one of New York's premier strategic law firms. The need for a fax machine operator was vital to our department at the time. Therefore, the description of the position went out to the recruitment agencies with immediate interviews following. I think Sherrell was the second or third applicant at that time. I remember it like it was yesterday. When she walked into the office, she carried a smile that brightened the entire room. Sherrell was beautiful, bright, adorable and hilarious all at the same time. Eventually, she was offered employment with our firm. And that's how we both met. After that, she was always "My Girl" Sherrell. We supported each other like sisters. We would visit each other's home and mingle with each other's family. We've shared good and bad times together.

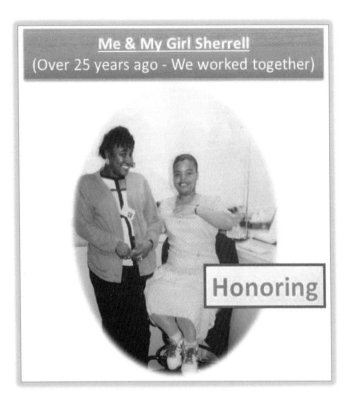

Me & My Girl Sherrell
(Over 25 years ago - We worked together)

Honoring

On one occasion when Sherrell visited me at my home, she would pick at my son NahDreams. She would give him kisses, which he had no problem accepting. She asked NahDreams, "Would you like to marry me when you grow up?" And NahDreams so innocently, replied "yes." Sherrell would then kiss and tickle him until he couldn't take it anymore.

On other occasions she would remind me to keep my good-looking son away from her daughters. Yeah, she had three beautiful little daughters just a few years younger than NahDreams. But today, everyone is all grown up and doing their own thing and Sherrell and I remained friends for a long time. *Amen.*

And as soon as I found out about my illness, I informed my loving and dear friend Sherrell. We would occasionally pray and talk on the phone to communicate with one another. She couldn't visit me at the time because she was helping to take care of her family. But she did make it her business to call me when she could. I always admired her for that — family values and all. A real woman — work, family, loyalty and love.

Unfortunately, a short while later, she was diagnosed with lung cancer. And here I was feeling devastated for *her*. Yet *she* wasn't; she assured me that everything was going to be all right. All I could do was be there for her as much as possible. I just wish I could've been there for her more.

The both of us facing the same fight and fighting it together blew our minds completely. I prayed to God that He would give me the strength to keep her spirits up — all while trying so desperately to keep up mine.

Unfortunately, we were living far apart from one another, with no Internet service on my end and our only form of quick communication was via telephone. And we have to thank God for that. *Amen.*

Meanwhile, a few months later, in May 2015, one setback led to another and My Girl Sherrell was gone. My sweet Sherrell was GONE from us — it happened so quickly — only God knows why. I will never forget the strength and positive attitude she possessed. How loving, supportive and considerate she was to her family and friends, especially her children (Kelvin, Shanique, Shakeera and Sharese) and eight grandchildren (Jaiden, Zhariyah, Khamayah, Amirah, Khalila, Khaliq, Darius and Deyana), with another grandchild on the way. May you all stay strong. Sherrell will always be in our hearts. *Amen.*

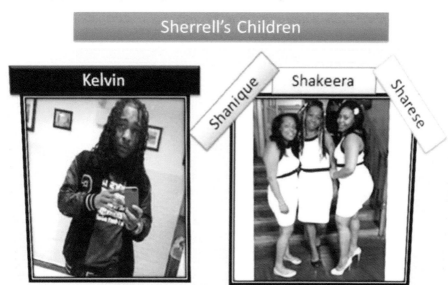

Sherrell's Children

Kelvin

Shanique

Shakeera

Sharese

Sherrell's Grandchildren

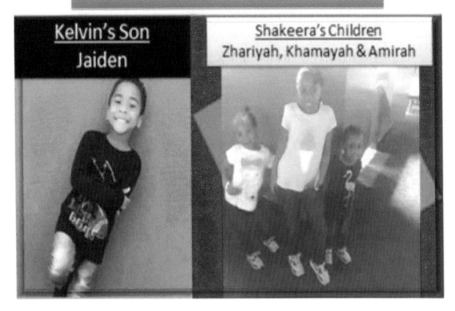

Kelvin's Son
Jaiden

Shakeera's Children
Zhariyah, Khamayah & Amirah

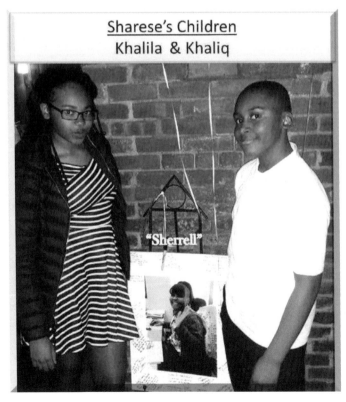

Sharese's Children
Khalila & Khaliq

Shanique's Children
Darius & Deyana

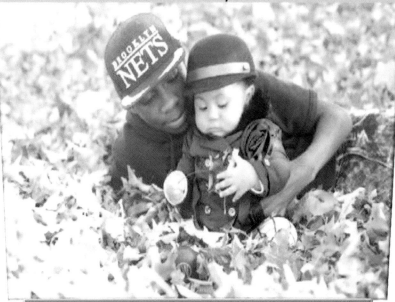

Just a few months prior to Sherrell's demise, her oldest daughter Shanique gave birth to a beautiful baby girl whom she named Deyana. At the time, not only was Deyana just born, but she was also Sherrell's *"8th Wonder of the World"*, and an adorable little replica of her as well. We've been blessed to have Deyana in our lives because through her, we've been given the opportunity to practically see Sherrell all over again. Wow! Every time Sherrell's children share pics and videos of the family, especially Deyana, I get emotional. So many fond memories flow right through me.

It's very rare to find an individual who you've shared over twenty-five years of friendship with. We don't get too many close friends like that in our lifetime, and I can assure you, Sherrell was definitely one of my closest friends. She will always be alive in my heart, as my best friend, and My Girl Sherrell!

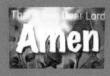

Every year on Facebook, I proudly pay tribute to My Girl Sherrell in honor of her birthday.

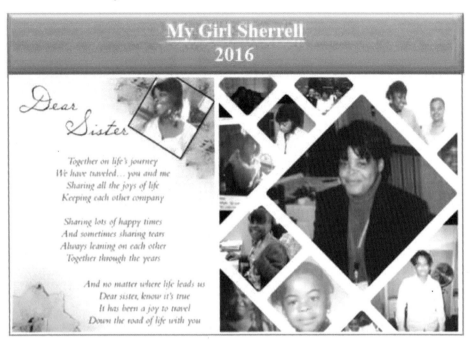

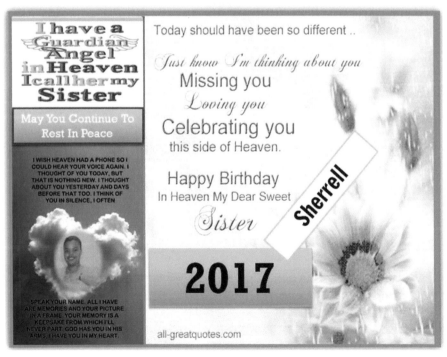

I've known Sherrell for a great number of years and can describe her in just five words: "A BLESSING TO HAVE KNOWN!" May you rest in peace my family, my friend, My Girl Sherrell.

Girlfriend Liza:

Liza and I worked together at the same company while living in South Carolina. We shared a lot of laughs together and both lived in the same hometown of Andrews. Since we were scheduled to work the same shift, Liza decided to start a carpool with all the staff members to split the cost of gas expenses when traveling to and from work. Liza was the designated driver and would never miss a day off from work. There were four of us in total and we could always count on Liza's loyalty and dedication.

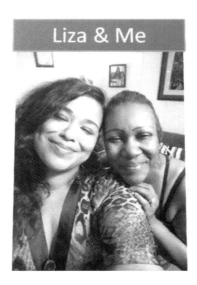

Liza & Me

But after only a few months of employment, I decided to move on. The position wasn't really my cup of tea. Since we no longer worked together, I now rarely saw Liza. It was only once in a while at the neighborhood supermarket we would run into each other. Eventually I landed a job in a fast food restaurant. And after a couple of years, Liza stopped by the fast food restaurant where I worked. She was shocked to see me there because she knew that wasn't my field of expertise. In any event, the expression on her face told it all. I recall her asking if I was all right. She mentioned to me how great I looked but she said it with uncertainty. I believe it was my weight loss that confused her. She wasn't used to seeing me so small and was a little concerned and worried. I informed her that I was ok but couldn't wait to get out of this kitchen. She knew exactly what I was talking about. *Amen.*

Shortly after, when she was informed of my illness, Liza would occasionally stop by my home to encourage me. We would talk, have laughs and enjoy each other's company. Ed would make us delicious dinners and we would sit back and enjoy them all. Liza's visits were most memorable to our family. She possesses brilliance, intelligence, wittiness, beauty and, being an outgoing kind of a person. She loves life and life loves her — and that's the type of attitude she has.

What I love about Liza the most is that she is from New York just like me. And when we worked at the same company, co-workers would call her Miss New York and we would just laugh. I didn't have a nickname at the time. I think Liza stood out more because of her fun-loving ways and approach on life. She has the most exciting personality. You could never get bored with her. She's just a good person to be around. *Amen.*

To Liza: Although we've only known one another for several years, you have become a very close and dear friend to me. On the days I was unable to get out of the house, you would always visit, and bring that big, beautiful and vibrant smile with you. I will always appreciate that. Thank you for being a dear friend and making my gloomy days brighter. God bless.

Girlfriend Charlene:

Charlene and I didn't meet until I moved to South Carolina. Interestingly, we shared the same birthday and were both associated with the same apartment complex as well as the fast food place of employment. Charlene always possessed a friendly warm-like welcoming smile to me. It appeared to me that my new name in the South was "Ms. Shirley". Now, although I'm from

New York I can get used to this "southern comfort," because here in the South, many people believe in addressing others by title, followed by first name. Culturally, that's the way it is done here in the South and I don't mind it at all since it's a form of respect.

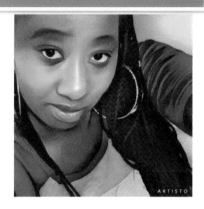

Girlfriend Charlene

On one occasion, I wasn't feeling too well but decided to accompany my husband to the grocery store anyway. While he shopped, I remained in the vehicle and waited. Shortly after, when he returned, he mentioned that he ran into my girlfriend Charlene and how she refused to let him pay for our food. So she paid for it and the price wasn't important at all. OMG. Wow! I was surprised, yet felt touched and grateful all at the same time. Unfortunately, I couldn't thank her until later. My health wasn't too well and I wasn't dressed appropriately at the time. But at the same time I was in shock, crying and felt so touched that someone with their own problems had time for me.

I mean, Charlene had four beautiful but busy kids, household expenses and a lot more on her plate to handle. So I don't understand how she was able to help me in my situation. She did know I was sick and struggling with this illness, and low on cash while working as a one-income household. But Charlene put on her I'm-gonna-help-Miss Shirley-hat and did what she wanted to do.

Lord, please bless Charlene and her family for her friendship, honesty, loyalty and faith in helping others. *Amen.*

Girlfriend Lewanda:

My very close girlfriend was informed immediately of my illness. She lived in New York during this time and was also experiencing poor health herself. Like me, she was unable to travel long distances. However, on occasion, she would call to check on the status of my health and my spirits. We would talk about the good old days and the many beautiful moments we shared together — like going to dance functions, vacationing, attending church functions, weddings and funerals. Lewanda always found a way to amuse me while at the same time keeping my spirits up.

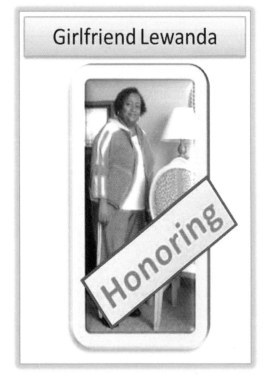

This wonderful woman and her husband Gregory have been close to our family for over 40 years. As best friends, she and I have shared a great deal of good and bad times together. Actually, Lewanda is related to my husband Ed as first cousins. Both of their mothers were related as sisters and that's what makes them first cousins.

On one occasion, my husband Ed and I were spending quality time together with Lewanda and Gregory, when all of a sudden, Lewanda was complaining about irritation in her back area. Immediately following, Gregory took her to the doctor's office for a checkup, and she was then diagnosed with shingles. The family was so sad to hear this news, that we rushed directly to the hospital, gathered in a circle, held each other's hand and prayed to God that she would pull through successfully. And yes, within time, she did make it through.

Thank you God for bringing my friend back to life and removing all of her pain and suffering. The devil was trying to make a way in but you sure showed him the way out. *Amen.*

However, after relocating to South Carolina, our close and long-time friendship took a turn for the worse and we landed in a blizzard of confusion. In hindsight, it should have never occurred, but it did. Actually, the confusion of our relationship was really all about nothing, and it was nothing worth losing a dear friend over. My move from New York to South Carolina left us distraught, devastated and depressed, so much that I created a poem in honor of our friendship, all while actually not even knowing where our friendship stood.

Forever Friends

Dedicated to LL

We were very close friends back in the day
And then we stopped speaking because of our selfish ways
But today, and every so often, we do talk
With occasional visits and frequent phone calls

Both of our families with so much in common
Became even closer than we could ever imagine
We'll never admit what really went wrong
But our special friendship is forever gone

We had our fun playing poker all night
Good times in Atlantic City until the morning light
We've been to many dances and parties together
We've been through the hurt, as well as the pleasure

But now we reminisce about the good and bad times
We spent them together consuming brandy and wine
The thoughts of these moments will never disappear
I refuse to forget, it would be more than I can bear

Forever in my heart, you will always be
The oldest and dearest friend to me
And with this in mind, friends are forever
Our relationship will last if we only endeavor

Shirley Valentine

A copy of the poem was sent to Lewanda and she fell in love with it right away because it was a heartfelt poem about our friendship. Lewanda always loved and respected my poems, and if she had any opinions about them she wouldn't hesitate to tell me so. In return, that's what I respected about her the most — her honesty.

Once Lewanda was told of my illness, she asked me if I wanted to pray with her, and, of course I did. Oh, how beautiful it was to hear her voice — soft but yet strong — to actually hear and feel my friend share my pain with me. I felt such contentment as she read. Was this an epiphany? I was actually releasing myself from all the pain and suffering I was enduring; my mind, body and soul were floating on a cloud as if I didn't have a care in the world. And after the first couple of prayer readings, she decided to send me the actual prayer booklet.

<u>Read & Pray & then Obey</u>
<u>by Lindsay Roberts</u>

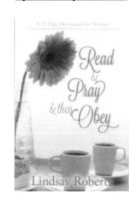

To know that someone cared for me was a blessing in itself. Not everybody can say that. My heart felt such love and happiness, and it was pure contentment when she read to me. I was so grateful to have an angel in my corner.

I thoroughly read the booklet and understood it to the fullest. I respect and appreciate anyone who shows others the Word of God. Lindsay Roberts' book has inspired me to get closer to my God. *Amen.*

To Lewanda: I am honoring you for the battle you won with your struggle with shingles. I saw you go through a very sad and painful period in her life, but with our prayers, we were fortunate to make it through a frightening and unbearable situation.

I want to thank you so much Lewanda for being a dear friend to me — for helping to make my life worth living. Your friendship as well as your prayers are the main reasons I am here today. May God always bless you and keep you safe. *Amen.*

Ms. Ruby:

Ms. Ruby was the mother of my best friend Lewanda. She was also the aunt of my husband Ed, because she and Ed's mother Ms. Lottie were siblings.

Ms. Ruby

Posted on FB – 7/1/16

Ms Ruby
So sad to say but today my 2nd MOM lost her battle with cancer and is finally resting with the lord She has been in pain for quite some time now I remember the love and prayers we shared through this entire ordeal You are truly missed by all I love you Ms Ruby sending prayers for her family and friends Amen

Posted on FB – 7/3/16

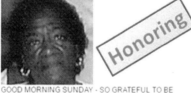

GOOD MORNING SUNDAY - SO GRATEFUL TO BE HERE ON THIS BEAUTIFUL DAY

Re Ms Ruby   (Lewanda's Mother) -- Thank you all for your condolences The Family and I are very grateful for the expressions of support we received from you all during such a difficult time

Ms. Ruby was very upset when she heard of my illness and insisted on supporting me by sending get well cards, prayers and money envelopes to help with my esteem. Although Ms. Ruby had been there for me in the past, this is the time that was most precious of all. And yet again, she was there for me. I give thanks to this beautiful individual. *Amen.*

Unfortunately, a little while later, Ms. Ruby was diagnosed with uterine cancer and passed away soon after, at the age of 81.

I've always considered this woman as a second mother. Ms. Ruby was devoted to living in God's way and taught her children and grandchildren the same. She will forever have a place in my heart and I will never forget her. What I respected about her the most was her belief in being there for family, no matter the situation, because God would make a way. *Amen.*

Grandma Nellie:

Grandma Nellie was born in October 1909 and raised in the South until adulthood. Eventually, looking for a better way of life, she relocated to New York where she continued to raise her family. Grandma Nellie was the mother of two daughters and one son. The oldest was Aunt Maggie, next was Momma, and then the youngest was Uncle Henry.

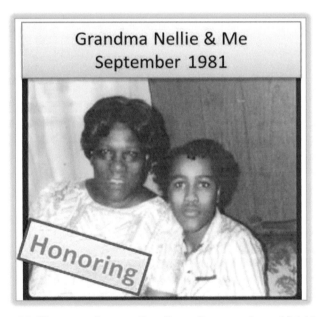

Grandma Nellie came from a fine line of strong, beautiful black women in her life. She and her three siblings were very close and lived in the same area of Brooklyn, NY. Ironically, Momma and Grandma Nellie's Momma had both raised four girls, and, Grandma Nellie's sisters were very special to us.

As young children, we would spend a great portion of time at Grandma Nellie's house. On many occasions, we would visit our grand aunts as well, by walking from one apartment complex to the other. We were very fortunate that they didn't live far apart from one another. Every visit was spent socializing and playing in front of their buildings, and there, we would play hopscotch, crazy eights, go fish, jump rope, and other popular games.

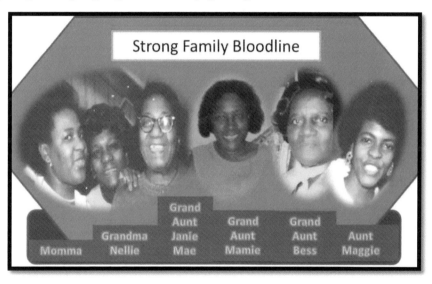

Our grand aunts enjoyed cooking, and when we came to visit, they would prepare delicious soul food meals just for us. It made us feel like it was Thanksgiving during every visit because we definitely had a lot to be grateful for. *Amen.*

Aunt Bess was a very sweet auntie, but at times, could be a hot mess. She loved to talk and always enjoyed having us kids over for visits. And, if you needed support, she would give you the shirt off of her back. But, if you gave her a hard way to go, she would raise her voice and threaten to knock you out, if she had to. At least that's what I witnessed! I remember once when we were visiting our grand aunts, Aunt Bess and Aunt Mamie were engaging in a little argument over the dimness of the lighting in the living room. Aunt Mamie thought maybe there wasn't enough lighting, so she decided to turn them on. But, when Aunt Bess saw what she had done, she demanded that Aunt Mamie turn the lights back off. But Aunt Mamie refused, and insisted that it was a little too dark for her. So, Aunt Bess decided to get a little aggressive and told her sister that if she was to turn the lights back on again, she was going to knock her out. Aunt Mamie decided then, to turn the other cheek as opposed to the lights being on. And if I could remember clearly, it was aunt Bess's home we were actually visiting during this time. So, you know we certainly didn't hear the last of that incident. *Amen.*

My beautiful grand aunts didn't always agree with one another — but they didn't hesitate in speaking their minds either. All the years spent as sisters, they've always looked out for one another, no matter what. And, when I look back on those days, I remember my grand aunts as being very respectable individuals who took pride in taking care of their loved ones.

Grand aunt Mamie gave birth to one son, and he is Momma's last surviving first cousin — Bill. Cousin Bill has a total of six children, eight grandchildren and seven great grandchildren with another one on the way. For 17 years, he has been married to a loving and dedicated woman — Elaine. Grand aunt Janie Mae had one son, Willie Bee, seven grandchildren and seven great grandchildren. Grand aunt Bess had one son, I-Jay, two granddaughters and several great grandchildren as well. *Amen.*

We used to get excited whenever Grandma Nellie came to visit as well. She would bring us graham crackers wrapped in paper plastic and give us each change or a $1.00 bill to carry to the corner grocery store for penny candy and other inexpensive items.

10

---

10 http://img.aws.livestrongcdn.com/ls-article-image-673/cme/cme_public_ images/www _livestrong_com/photos.demandstudios.com/getty/article/190/123/101195570_XS.jpg

We spent a lot of great times with Grandma Nellie as she did the same with us. *Amen!* One thing I will always remember about Grandma Nellie was her life stories. Some of her stories I just so happened to have witnessed myself:

It was a cold winter day and Grandma Nellie came to spend some time with our family. After her visit she would let us, the grands visit her at her home for the weekend. She lived in Fort Greene, Brooklyn and traveling to her home consisted of riding on the bus and train. And on this specific weekend, I was the chosen one.

The bus stop was the very first step to getting to Grandma Nellie's house. Well, there we were, in the cold, on a breezy day and waiting for the neighborhood bus. Not much later, we could see the bus a couple of blocks away. Grandma Nellie decides to take her canister of snuff out prior to getting on the bus. So she raises the snuff up to her mouth and places it under her bottom lip to take a dose. Then she starts her usual sucking all while the bus is getting closer and closer to our stop. At this point she knows she has to spit out the snuff because it's getting too strong to keep in her mouth. So now, she decides to spit it out right before the bus reaches our bus stop. Unfortunately, the wind was blowing so hard that the snuff, which was now in the form of mud, sadly landed on a man's light colored pants. OMG! The only thing I can remember is that he was so upset with Grandma Nellie. Prior to getting on the bus he did make a statement as to: "Hey lady, you just spit on me and messed up my pants" — something to that effect. Grandma Nellie was apologetic and felt so embarrassed that she hurried us both onto the bus. Actually, the man that got sprayed with the snuff, wind up not taking the bus after all. I guess after Grandma Nellie got finished "redecorating" his outfit, he had to go back home to change. Sorry about that fellow. Believe me, Grandma Nellie never meant any harm. *Amen.*

The train was the next step to getting to Grandma Nellie's house. It was the same exact day and Grandma Nellie wanted to know why people were staring at her. I was asleep when this all began but when I awoke, she was so upset that she had to express her feelings to me. I took one look at her and realized that she was wearing only one eye lens in her glasses. I had no other choice but to give her the news. So she took her index finger and placed it near the first eye, but that wasn't the correct eye. She then used the same procedure for the other eye and wind up, poking herself right in the socket. Lord, have mercy. That was an experience I'll never forget. The second time around, almost took Grandma Nellie's eye out. I felt bad about her eye but also, couldn't contain myself from this comical matter. God bless you Grandma Nellie.

The final step to getting to Grandma Nellie's house was the second, but final bus ride. Based on what we just experienced, all we could do was laugh and hug each other through the entire ride. These moments were the most memorable moments ever experienced with Grandma Nellie.

Grandma Nellie was a strong, direct and no-nonsense type of woman. She was a Christian woman, and although she may have sipped on the yak, mingled in her favorite peach snuff and enjoyed drinking beer, she didn't take any mess from anyone, especially my Pop.

As an adolescent, I recall one occasion when Momma was admitted into the hospital for a procedure. Grandma Nellie had agreed to babysit and was in charge of the household funds. But, just like old school, she had a habit of keeping her money in a small black purse, located close to her bosom. Well, one night she went to sleep and the following morning when she awoke, her little black purse was located right beside her and empty at that. Of course, Pop was nowhere to be found. But thank goodness Grandma Nellie made a way and we were back on our feet again. I'm not quite sure how she did it, but she did it. *Amen.*

Grandma Nellie had a habit of constantly talking in a loud tone, and when Pop was around, it would drive him crazy. So, on another occasion, I witnessed my Grandma Nellie and Pop going at it. Grandma Nellie came over for a visit and Pop couldn't hear the TV because she was talking too loud. He would ask her to lower her voice, but he would ask her in a cruel and nasty way. But Grandma Nellie caught on to his sneaky ways and continued to talk, and at a higher volume this time. He would then walk over to the TV set and turn the volume up in order to tune her out. Again, Grandma Nellie wouldn't give in. She would continue to raise the tone of her voice until Pop couldn't take it anymore. Pop would say some naughty words back to Grandma Nellie, hoping that she would go back home. But then, she would say to Pop: "You can turn the TV up if you want, but I'm not going anywhere." Eventually, at the end of the day, Pop would give up first. Grandma Nellie's constant and loud talking always seemed to outweigh and outlast anything he threw her way. She would run him right out of the living room and directly into another.

Unfortunately, later in her years, Grandma Nellie was diagnosed with diabetes and gangrene, and it had gotten so severe that, eventually, one of her legs had to be amputated. Shortly after, the other leg needed to be amputated as well and she had to wear prosthetic legs and carry a cane. At times, when she would remove her prosthetic legs for comfort, we would go and sit by her side to

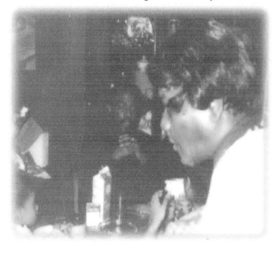

massage, jiggle and sometimes just flap the bottom of her knees back and forth, because they felt so much like jelly.

Family moments were shared wisely while sitting at the dinner table together. We used to keep ourselves busy by eating snacks, playing cards or board games or, just enjoying one another's company. Sometimes Grandma Nellie would pace slowly through the house, moving from room to room and talking all while praising the Lord. I wonder what my brother David had on his mind at that time. God bless you Grandma Nellie and may you continue to rest in peace. *Amen.*

Aunt Maggie:

Aunt Maggie was Momma's older sister. She was bright, beautiful, smart and charming. Unfortunately, lung cancer took her life in her early 50s. It was so devastating for our family. Though it felt as if it happened so quickly, she had actually been ill for some time. Aunt Maggie was the strong-willed aunt who paved the way for others. She designed and created her own costume jewelry as well as her own clothing line. She also sold Avon products to help supplement her income. Her ability to be creative and make people happy was a God-sent blessing.

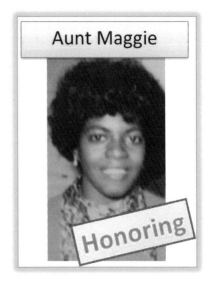

When we were little, our aunt actually created and sewed our dresses for school portrait day. My baby sister and I had the same look that school year. I was in the third grade and she was in the first grade. Sister Gail wore her hair

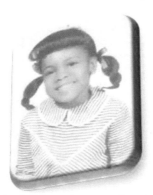

with a big beautiful curly bang and two twisted ponytails, and with big bright green ribbons to match. Our dresses were very much similar but made a little differently around the neck.

129

For me, Aunt Maggie made a pretty green and white-striped dress with lace trimming around the neck. It also had lace trim from one shoulder down to

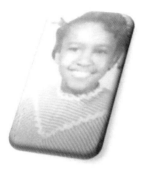

the mid-chest area and up again to the other shoulder, forming a V-neck. To top off, Momma tied a big bright green ribbon on the top right side of my hair. I was off to school and a happy child I was — *Amen.*

I was in the fifth grade when my aunt helped to buy my clothes for that year's portrait day as well. This white ruffled long-sleeve shirt made me feel like an adult. It had a red lining along the trim and it was pressed to a Tee. And along with that joyful smile, it was a day to remember.

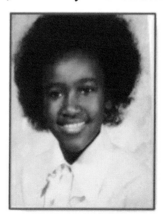

All of the kids wanted to believe I was wearing a wig and they proceeded to tease me just about every day. But the hair was all mine and I couldn't convince them any differently. On many occasions, I would come home from school, run into my bedroom and cry myself to sleep. I'm just glad I didn't become a scorned individual today because of the bullying. Thank you God. *Amen.*

As a young girl — I can't quite remember the age — but my first bicycle came from this very same woman. And when it was time to remove the training wheels, I practically felt like I became an adult. My older brother Steven assisted me with that one. RIP Brother. I remember so well how he insisted I not look back while he was pushing me on my bike. I was riding way down the street thinking he had my back just in case I would fall. But after pedaling for a couple of minutes, I turned around and saw him way down the street where we actually began. OMG! I was so upset. So, of course, I fell off of my bike. My confidence level went downtown. I knew what he was trying to do, but I just couldn't believe his dishonesty. In any event, I got over it and became a pretty good bike rider. *Amen.*

In this photo Sis. Linda was about 13 years of age when Aunt Maggie created this beautiful jumpsuit for her. My younger sister was stepping out on this day — just styling and profiling. It was Easter Sunday, and we usually enjoyed this holiday by spending it with close family and friends. *Amen.*

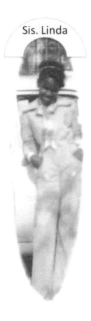

Sis. Linda

It was the summer of 1975 and time for me to take middle school portrait photos. By this time the afro was gone, the curls were in and the teasing of the afro disappeared. And although the afro was the hairdo folks wore at the time, I decided to go with the curls. Just didn't want to deal with any more teasing. I was about to graduate from middle school with honors, especially in typing. So, it was time to get myself together for school portrait day. My only dilemma was that Momma had no idea what outfit I was going to wear. So she asked my aunt to help us out, and as usual, Aunt Maggie was there to rescue us again. Aunt Maggie loved her only sister so much that she would do practically anything to please her.

Wow! My hair was long and shiny with real big curls starting with the bang, and working itself around to the back of my neck, and ending up on the other side of my head. Although the blouse was store-bought, the pantsuit was created by my Aunt 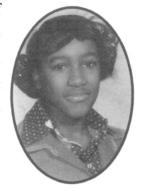 Maggie. It was bright red and full of potential. The jacket had a small square pocket on the left hand side of the chest and a white double knit stitch around the collar. The pants had two pockets, one on each side, buttons in front, and a crease that stood tall. I was a bad mamma jamma on that day!

During this time in my life, I wasn't quite sure what my future career would hold. But I did have a sense that it would involve some form of typing. After all, I was the fastest typist in my class while enjoying it all at the same time. On many occasions, other students and I would compete with one another in testing one's ability, and I always managed to come out first. Hope you girls can remember me! *Amen.*

As a teenager, my aunt asked me if I would be interested in attending sewing classes for the summer. I thought that was a great idea because I'd seen and had worn the clothes that she designed. And if my aunt can show me what she knows, then I'm all for it.

I'll never forget when she sent my cousin Sharon and me to sewing classes for the summer. Sharon was Aunt Maggie's daughter and my first cousin and we were very close. And lucky little ladies we were. By bus, we only lived about a half-hour away from the sewing class which was also located in Jamaica, Queens. We had a lot of fun attending classes together and were very excited to have made our first outfit. You must first start out with a pattern which is the

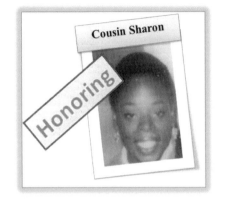

Cousin Sharon

template from which the parts of a garment are traced onto fabric before being cut out and assembled. We decided to make a pantsuit with a vest and no jacket. And, yes, the pants had side pockets and a zipper. We were so proud that we could make clothing if we needed to.

Unfortunately, my cousin Sharon passed away from colon cancer while in her mid-30s. She was a loving and beautiful individual. We shared so many laughs as well as cries together and I miss her dearly. So, on this day, I am honoring you for your fight and struggle with cancer. May you rest in peace Cousin Sharon. *Amen.*

It was June 1979 and time to take photos again, but this time it was for my high school graduation. I recall vaguely, that on this occasion, something distraught had occurred that would change our lives forever.

Aunt Maggie had passed away prior to my graduation, and sadly, taking photos for this occasion didn't feel quite the same. I always wore and took

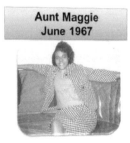

Aunt Maggie
June 1967

pride in what she had created for me in the past, so being unable to wear her creation on this special occasion was depressing for me. This was our day and she was always there for these memorable moments and now she wasn't.

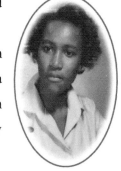

Prior to the deadline for taking my graduation photos, Momma and I went to the mall to purchase a beautiful new blouse to match my outfit. I was pleased with the blouse and wore it with pride and dignity in honor of my auntie.

I am honoring you, Aunt Maggie from up above. My aunt was a blessing (and not "in disguise") because everyone knew of her loving and giving ways. You will always be loved and missed. May you continue to rest in peace Auntie. *Amen.*

Uncle Henry:

Uncle Henry was Momma's only brother and he was also the youngest of her and Aunt Maggie. Uncle Henry had one daughter (Pamela) and one son (Darrell). Pamela has three children and three grandchildren. Darrell has six children and three grandchildren. We were very close, and today, still remain a tight family.

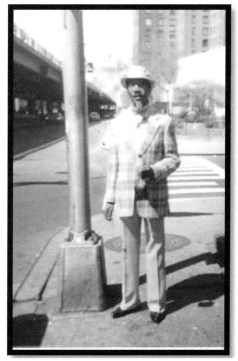

Uncle Henry resided in Fort Greene, Brooklyn where his mother Nellie used to live and subsequent to Grandma Nellie's death, he took over her apartment and lived there until his death. The way he carried himself, his character and appearance took on a certain persona of a "Mack Daddy." He was, however, the total opposite. Uncle

Henry just liked to play such a role because back then, it was the cool way to be. He wore a gray beard and a goatee to match. If you didn't know him you would say he was a straight-up hustler, akin to Antonio Fargas of *Starsky and Hutch*. While he may have rocked his wide-brim pimp daddy hat, old school plaid jacket and deep creases in his pants, he was a cool cat, who hustled in life in order to succeed. I remember him as being a good man to his nieces and nephews and a loving brother to my mother.

To help supplement his income, Uncle Henry would sell snow cones with flavored syrup. I may have been an adult at the time but I enjoyed Uncle Henry's snow cones. I used to love visiting him and standing over his mini truck, as he scraped the ice and placed it so lovingly into my cup. He would then add multiple flavored syrups to top it off. There was nothing like getting a taste of Uncle Henry's snow cones. There were plenty of times he wouldn't even charge me a cent. God bless his soul.

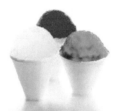

Uncle Henry would constantly remind us of his generosity though, as to when he would give us pocket change as kids. We were always grateful and today, we still are. As nieces and nephews, we would, of course, reciprocate. When Uncle Henry would visit us and vice versa, we would give him a few dollars to help him out. *Amen.*

One day, Uncle Henry invited me, my husband Ed, and Momma over for the day. When we arrived, he had a large painting of a topless woman hanging on the living room wall. Momma didn't respond and neither did I nor Ed. We just couldn't believe that Uncle Henry had the audacity to keep that painting on the wall while we visited. Momma believed that her brother knew better and so did I. I guess he felt it shouldn't have bothered us so much because we were

135

adults. But that wasn't the point. Where was the respect for women? Even Ed, as a man, was feeling out of place. We really didn't want to be around any type of nudity, especially in the presence of Momma. That alone was downright disrespectful. Well, we visited for a short while without saying a word about the painting, and then Ed eventually drove us back home. The visit turned out to be good after all, because we decided to just look the other way. *Amen.*

Unfortunately, in 2010 Uncle Henry passed away a few years after Pop. He exhibited a certain flair about himself, and showed a lot of pizazz in his everyday life. You will be truly missed Uncle Henry. May you rest in peace. *Amen.*

Cousin Bill:

Although Cousin Bill and Pop were very close, Cousin Bill was actually Momma's first cousin and both of their mothers (Mamie & Nellie) were sisters. Yet, Cousin Bill and Pop were like brothers at heart and ironically, shared the same last name. They've known each other for years and shared many memories since the late '40s.

On the day of Pop's passing, Cousin Bill was there for support. From what I understand, they were both spending the weekend in Atlantic City and shared the same hotel room. At one point, Pop had complained to Cousin Bill about severe back pains and, shortly thereafter, an ambulance was called to the casino. When they arrived, Pop was still alive and was then taken to the hospital. Once there, doctors worked on Pop for a short while to revive him, but to no avail. It was that time again. Another member of the family was gone. This had to be one of the most devastating scenes ever for Cousin Bill. When he explained to our family what had occurred, I was called immediately at my job and rushed home. Cousin Bill was distraught and in shock over the entire situation because Pop meant a great deal to him. To actually see a close family member be there one minute, and gone the next, had to be a frightening experience.

There was one summer vacation when Pop, Cousin Bill and Uncle Henry went to Georgia to visit family. When they returned home, they couldn't wait to share their experiences with us. You would think they were kids all over again. I guess that's how the South made them feel when they would visit. After all, Georgia was their home state, and this is where they grew up.

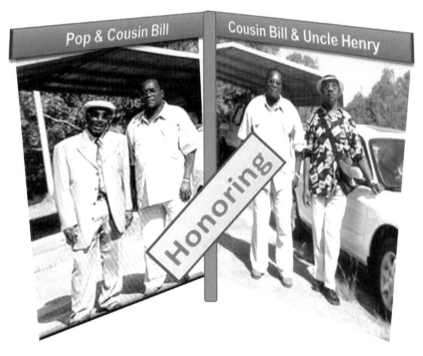

To Cousin Bill: I'm grateful to you, Cousin Bill, for being in the right place, and at the right time for Pop. You were also there for Uncle Henry as well and that makes you "double the man". I am honoring you for all the times you have been there for our family. Thanks for being you, and may God bless always. *Amen.*

Cousin Bill is currently 87 years of age, but when he was in his early 70s, he was diagnosed with arthritis and prostate cancer, and had to receive radiation and other medical treatments. He also had difficulties with his hips, but they were eventually replaced surgically on two separate occasions, which he also overcame. Thank you God. Cousin Bill is a very strong man who has fought so many obstacles in his life. His determination to overcome them has led to victories of success in healing of the body. But today, arthritis continues to be a burden on Cousin Bill. He does, however, continue to address it by taking medication and other remedies. *Amen.*

Cousin Deborah:

Cousin Deborah is Bill's daughter and my second cousin. Her grandma and my grandma were sisters and it just so happens that she and my brother David were born only one day apart. *Amen.*

Cousin Deborah has been blessed to have a wonderful, charming and dedicated spouse (Carl), who can cook his tail off, a beautiful and vivacious daughter (Tahisha) with a highly talented singing voice, an intelligent and handsome son (Ahlyjus) who has recently graduated from college, and an incredibly highly talented and good-looking grandson (Makiah) who is also Tahisha's son.

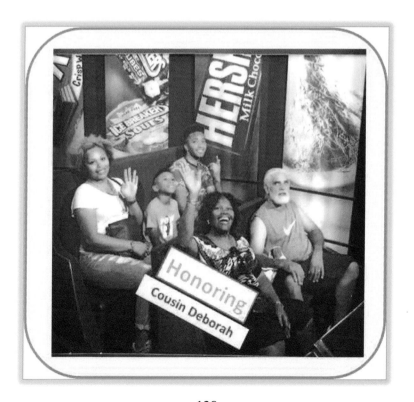

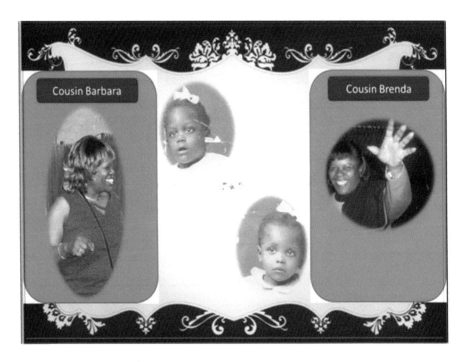

Barbara, Brenda and Randy are also Cousin Bill's children, and happily, my second cousins. While these beautiful ladies are the middle siblings, Randy is the baby boy of the family. You all have shown so much love and support by keeping up with the progress of my health and also by interacting with me on Facebook's video chat.

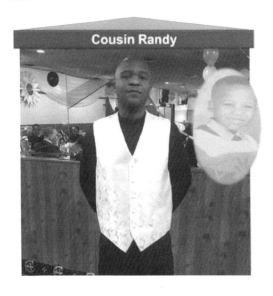

Michael is Cousin Bill's oldest child and my second cousin as well. He and Momma's oldest son Terry were born the same year.

Michael and his wife Audrey do their best in keeping up with the faces of technology on Facebook. I am very proud of my family for showing me love and support throughout my entire life. I will always be grateful to you all.

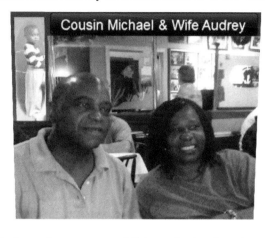

Cousin Michael & Wife Audrey

Jenelle is Cousin Bill's sixth and youngest child, and she has just celebrated her sixteenth birthday with close family, friends and schoolmates. Happy Birthday Cousin Jenelle! Cousin Jenelle is being accompanied by her mom Elaine as they approach the stage to address their family and friends for sharing in this spectacular event together. *Amen.*

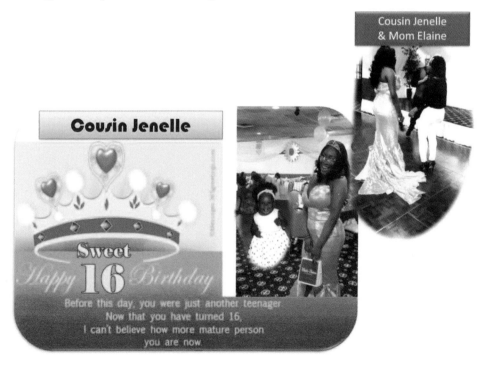

Cousin Jenelle & Mom Elaine

Cousin Jenelle

Sweet Happy 16 Birthday

Before this day, you were just another teenager.
Now that you have turned 16,
I can't believe how more mature person
you are now.

Cousin Jenelle is currently in high school with plans to attend college while majoring in music, and with dreams of becoming a future performer or music director. We all love you. May you continue to grow and mature into a beautiful and intelligent woman. *Amen.*

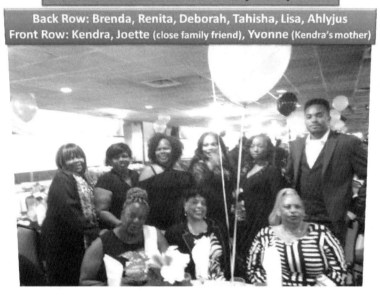

Jenelle's Sweet 16th Birthday Party Bash

Back Row: Brenda, Renita, Deborah, Tahisha, Lisa, Ahlyjus
Front Row: Kendra, Joette (close family friend), Yvonne (Kendra's mother)

I know I haven't actually seen this side of my family for some years, but hopefully through prayers, we will all meet again real soon. Thanks Deborah, Barbara and Michael for providing two more generations of our family legacy. Our children will be provided with more opportunity of learning about our family's history. Thank you all for being great cousins and for also keeping up with the technology of the world. How else were we going to actually stay in touch with each other? Facebook has

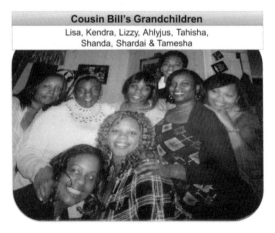

Cousin Bill's Grandchildren
Lisa, Kendra, Lizzy, Ahlyjus, Tahisha, Shanda, Shardai & Tamesha

made a difference in our lives and we should never take it for granted. Thanking God for such a creation has definitely given my life a whole new meaning. *Amen!*

To Cousin Deborah: When you found out about my illness, you immediately collaborated with other family members and came to my rescue. And although you weren't involved in Facebook at the time, you did manage to communicate through other sources and put a smile on my face. Keeping up with the progress of my health was one of the most touching experiences one cousin can give to another. You're the best Cousin Deborah and I will always be grateful to you.

Growing up, we learned a lot from you and your siblings. But you taught me and my sisters the meaning of "true beauty." You always made certain that

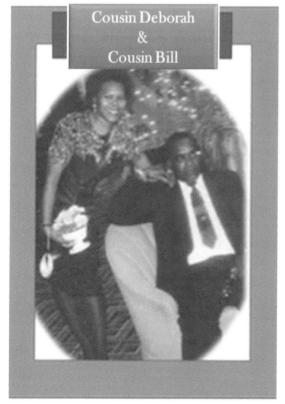

Cousin Deborah
&
Cousin Bill

we understood that beauty is in the eye of the beholder and to not judge people based on their exterior. We admired you then, and we admire you now for continuing to believe and teach the same to others.

On one occasion, during my teenage years, Cousin Deborah would take me to her bedroom and lead me directly into her walk-in closet. At that time, we wore roughly the same size clothing. Once there, she would slowly go through her wardrobe. While searching, she passes me one article of clothing. She searches again, and then, passes me another piece of clothing. Mind you, talking, all while searching for the articles of clothing she wanted me to have. I refused to say or interrupt my beautiful cousin in any way because she was on a roll, and the articles I would receive were sometimes new, and if not, were in excellent condition. Either way you look at it, I took pride in wearing all the beautiful clothing I received from Cousin Deborah. She was very generous and never hesitated to share her things. As young girls we found Cousin Deborah's wardrobe to be intriguing, colorful and yet, full of wear, if we could've helped it. LOL. She would give me denim jeans, blouses and sometimes jackets. Her clothes were always clean and pressed nicely; placed on hangers and ready to wear. I used to love wearing her denim jeans because the majority of them were bleached and during those times, this was in fashion.

I believe Cousin Deborah understood our family's situation — how Momma was struggling to make ends meet. But she didn't just roll over and play dead — she took action and provided her little cousins with a little something extra. This was her way of saying "I love you all." *Amen.*

On one occurrence, when Cousin Deborah and I were upstairs putting together my new wardrobe, my sisters Gail and Linda were downstairs standing by the closet door and doing a little modeling for the cameras. Immediately following that little vogue episode, they would quickly hang up their jackets and head straight for the door. And that's exactly what my sisters did, cut loose outside to spend some quality time with the neighborhood friends.

Cousin Bill also owned a miniature pool table which we all enjoyed playing. The table was located downstairs in the basement where he kept a number of games. I remember my brother Steven loved playing on this pool table and he would play it with class — in his self-made pantsuit. That's correct! Steven learned how to sew, and at times, would create unique outfits to wear on special occasions.

There were also times when I managed to follow my sisters' same example. Once getting to Cousin Bill's house, I would say my hellos, and head outside to see my neighborhood friends and classmates as well. There, I was able to share homework studies and fun times together when visiting. Thank God Cousin Bill didn't live too far away from my school. *Amen.*

I still reminiscence about those electrifying visits to Cousin Bill's house. We were always overly excited about visiting because there was something interesting happening during every stay. Whether it was a barbeque, birthday party or other special events, Cousin Bill's house was the place to be.

I am honoring you Cousin Deborah for making your little cousins feel more like sisters. I will love you endlessly. May God bless you. Thank you Cousin Bill for everything! *Amen.*

As a family, we would sometimes meet up and share some laughs together. Actually, the last time we got together with the family was in July 2010 in Atlantic City. I'll never forget how you guys came to see Ed and me that weekend for our anniversary celebration. We, as a family, enjoyed each other's company and shared lots of fond memories on this wonderful and blessed trip.

Ed, Me, Bill, Renita, Deborah & Linda

I pray that Ed and I will have the opportunity to share more beautiful times with our family. God bless. *Amen.*

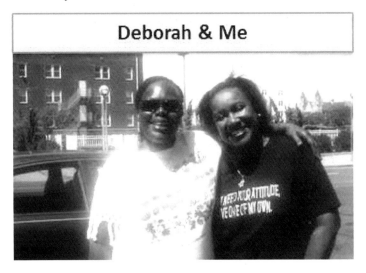

Aunt Sara:

Aunt Sara is Big Naheen's aunt and the older sister of his father Billy. She is currently 80 years young, and beautiful as ever. I met Aunt Sara in 1979 through my relationship with Big Naheen. Her side of the family would call him "Junior".

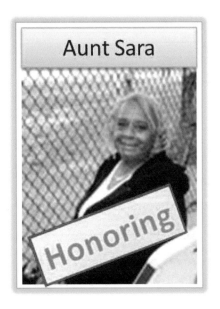

To Aunt Sara: When you found out about my illness, you would talk and pray with me via telephone. While you were in the middle of your own storm, you paused to help provide me with love, support and prayer through mine. Just knowing that you've been through two knee replacements and one elbow replacement is too much to bear, but I'm so glad you made it through successfully. I do continue to pray that your health is blessed with only the good in life, and that your fight with rheumatoid disease, disappears forever.

I have always admired you for showing concern for others no matter what. Obviously, God has given you the strength to do what you do best. *Amen.*

When Junior passed away, Aunt Sara was there to support me in my difficult time. Your being there when I was feeling so alone and vulnerable, meant the world to me. Thanks to you and your determination, together, we were successful in finding the support we needed so desperately to handle the affairs for Junior's departure. I want to thank Aunt Sara for being there for me through all of my times, happy and sad. I will always love you and God bless. *Amen.*

Father-in-law Billy:

My father-in-law Billy passed away in September, 1995 and will be missed forever. He was there for me, NahDreams and his son, Junior when we were down on our luck. I remember vaguely how huge his house was and how nicely it was decorated with wall-to-wall carpeting and layered with black shag throughout. I used to travel to work with his girlfriend Lois and her sister, and we shared some fun times on the subways and buses together.

At times, Billy would have to give his son, Junior some advice on life and what to say and not to say to women. On many occasions, Junior found ways of getting on my nerves and at times, I would have to involve his father. Although my father-in-law gave pretty good advice, sometimes Junior would let his father's advice go through one ear, and out the other. And that was Junior's way — at times, he could be very stubborn.

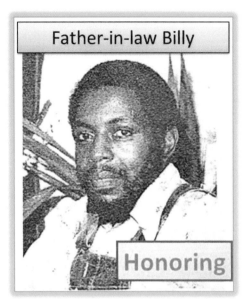

Father-in-law Billy

Honoring

Today, I am honoring you, my father-in-law Billy, from up above. I want to thank you for your strength and courage in being a strong individual who's always been known to give good advice to the younger generation. And although you and your son Junior didn't always agree on everything, he always loved you dearly. May you continue to rest in peace. *Amen.*

Aunt Linda:

Aunt Linda is Junior's aunt and the youngest sibling of both Sara and Billy. Aunt Linda and I met during the same time Aunt Sara and I was introduced. Back then, I would visit the family often, and we would relish in playing cards and board games together. And later, when NahDreams was born, Aunt Linda and the family would spoil him rotten to the core. My son was never alone and loved to be around Aunt Linda and her daughters (Evette and Monica). Later, Aunt Linda had a son and named him David, and until this day, NahDreams and I continue to remain close to them all. *Amen.*

When you found out about my illness you were distraught. Our connection has always been more like a big sister-little sister type of relationship. I know my drastic news was hard for you to handle because you knew, and still know, some of the consequences of carrying a deadly disease.

In the early 2000s, sadly, you were diagnosed with Lupus and the family was shocked to hear the news. Over the years, you've been suffering a great deal with this illness. But today, through the grace of God, you are currently in the stage of remission.

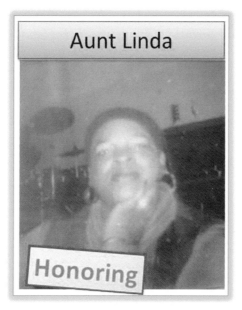

To Aunt Linda: Today and every day, I am honoring you for your bravery and strength in fighting your battle with Lupus. You are a strong, beautiful and radiant woman with the light of God shining upon you. May you continue to be blessed and may your sickness never return. *Amen.*

Aunt Bessie and Uncle Vince:

Aunt Bessie and Uncle Vince are the last living siblings on Pop's side of the family. There were a total of 8 children. Aunt Bessie is currently 97 years old and continues to carry the spunk of the vibrant young woman she once was. She is the eldest of the children and loves her brother Vince unconditionally. Uncle Vince is the baby brother of the family and is currently 83 years of age. To keep himself going strong, he often visits his older sister in a nursing home to share some good laughs and to make certain she has the necessities needed in her daily life. *Amen.*

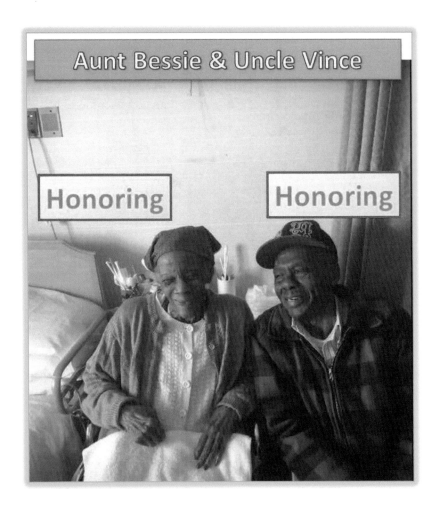

To Aunt Bessie and Uncle Vince: I am honoring the both of you for the warmth and strength that you provided to me during my lifetime. All the love, good times and bad times that we shared with Pop were most memorable, especially those days when we all would go to Atlantic City where we would stay up all night, just enjoying each other's company. Aunt Bessie, when you lived with me in the past, I would take notes on some of your dance moves. May you continue to shake your tail feather just like you used to do, back in the day. *Amen.* Uncle Vince, you sent me a warm and heartfelt envelope that contained lots of love and support. May you continue to smile and share lots of laughs and love with the family. *Amen.*

149

Cousin Cynthia:

Cynthia is Aunt Janie Mae's granddaughter and my second cousin. Both of our grandmothers were sisters. Cousin Cynthia has two children: the oldest is Michael, the youngest is Kevin.

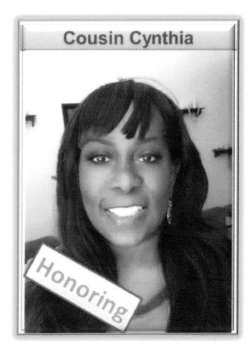

We haven't been in touch with one another for quite some time now, but recently, I had the pleasure of communicating with my cousin. Although she isn't familiar with Facebook, we were able to reach out to one another through telephone and e-mail. Some of us don't have an account with Facebook, and prefer to use other forms of social media. Whichever way is effective in reaching out to a loved one, is fine by me. Even though we haven't been in touch for a while, we enjoyed a deep conversation about our family memories, current situations, and of course, our future destinies.

Unfortunately though, Cousin Cynthia was diagnosed with liver cancer in 2010, and today, is still fighting this disease. At one point, the cancer was gone, but later, had returned. Cousin Cynthia is currently going through radiation treatments and other treatments to help resolve the cancer.

To Cousin Cynthia: Today, and every day, I honor you for your fight and struggle with liver cancer. I hope and pray that you overcome this fight so that your journey in life is clearer. May all your pain disappear, and be replaced with nothing but love and joy. I love you Cousin Cynthia, always and forever. God bless. *Amen.*

It is a tremendous honor to pay tribute to the living, as well as the deceased. God, I love my family. *Amen.*

Other Family & Friends:

Other family and friends were really never told of my illness and if they were, it was only because they were very close to us.

I would like to thank my family for allowing me to share their health issues with you all. I would also like to thank all of my family and friends for loving and supporting me in my fight with cancer. God bless. *Amen.*

CHAPTER 10. CHEMOTHERAPY TREATMENTS & MCLEOD BADGE OF COURAGE AWARD

Unfortunately, my first scheduled chemotherapy treatment was rescheduled due to my high blood pressure. That's pretty normal for me because high blood pressure runs in my family. But, it really isn't cool having high blood pressure; it's a very serious disease that can lead to death. And, at best, it can cause other medical problems that can eventually prevent you from living an everyday normal life. So please people, don't wait to get high blood pressure by ignoring the signs. Avoid getting it by eating right, exercising, dieting, physical checkups and, of course, maintaining a relationship with God. It also wouldn't hurt to purchase your own blood pressure monitor. Today, keeping track of my blood pressure is extremely important for my health.

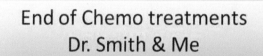

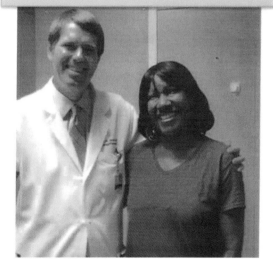

Once my blood pressure stabilized to an acceptable level, my doctor rescheduled my chemotherapy treatments. Through the grace of God, I completed them all.

Chemotherapy Appts.
3/27/14 - Rescheduled for 4/3/14
1st - 4/3/14
2nd - 4/24/14
3rd - 5/15/14
4th - 6/5/14
5th - 6/26/14
6th - 7/17/14

McLeod Badge of Courage Award

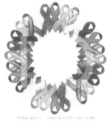

McLeod Badge
of
Courage Award

This is to certify that

Shirley Valentine

Has completed chemotherapy

On this day, the __17th__ of _July_, _2014_

Signed: _Annette_
McLeod Cancer Center

Don't get me wrong, it was extremely difficult and emotional to make it through the process of recovery. However, sometimes in life, especially times like this, we don't have much of a choice if we want to fight for our lives. Thank you God for keeping me strong through this entire ordeal. *Amen.*

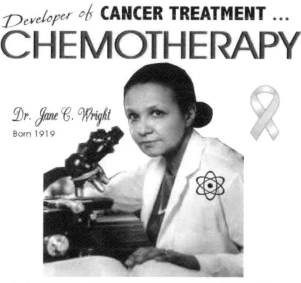

Developer of **CANCER TREATMENT ...**

CHEMOTHERAPY

Dr. Jane C. Wright
Born 1919

Dr. Jane Wright and her father Dr. Louis T. Wright (1891 ~ 1952)
discovered and developed chemicals that attack and destroy cancer
cells called chemotherapeutic agents. An effective treatment for most
forms of cancer today.

www.blackmiracles.com

Achievements:

1971: Dr. Jane Wright was the first woman to be elected president of the
New York Cancer Society.

1967: Dr. Jane Wright became professor of surgery, head of the cancer
chemotherapy department, and associate dean at New York Medical College, and
the highest ranked African American woman at a nationally recognized medical
institution.

Inspiration:

Jane Cooke Wright's father was one of the first African American
graduates of Harvard Medical School, and he set a high standard for his
daughters. Dr. Louis Wright was the first African American doctor appointed to a

---

[11] See more: https://cfmedicine.nlm.nih.gov/physicians/biography_336.html

staff position at a municipal hospital in New York City and, in 1929, became the city's first African American police surgeon. He also established the Cancer Research Center at Harlem Hospital. Jane Wright graduated with honors from New York Medical College in 1945.

Louis Tompkins Wright

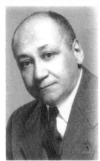

Biography:

Dr. Jane Wright analyzed a wide range of anti-cancer agents, explored the relationship between patient and tissue culture response, and developed new techniques for administering cancer chemotherapy. By 1967, she was the highest ranking African American woman in a United States medical institution.

Born in New York City in 1919, Jane Cooke Wright was the first of two daughters born to Corrine (Cooke) and Louis Tompkins Wright. Her father was one of the first African American graduates of Harvard Medical School, and he set a high standard for his daughters. Dr. Louis Wright was the first African American doctor appointed to a staff position at a municipal hospital in New York City and, in 1929, became the city's first African American police surgeon. He also established the Cancer Research Center at Harlem Hospital.

Jane Wright graduated with honors from New York Medical College in 1945. She interned at Bellevue Hospital from 1945 to 1946, serving nine months as an assistant resident in internal medicine. While completing a residency at Harlem Hospital from 1947 to 1948, she married David Jones, Jr., a Harvard Law School graduate. After a six-month leave for the birth of her first child in 1948, she returned to complete her training at Harlem Hospital as chief resident.

155

In January 1949, Dr. Wright was hired as a staff physician with the New York City Public Schools, and continued as a visiting physician at Harlem Hospital. After six months she left the school position to join her father, director of the Cancer Research Foundation at Harlem Hospital.

Chemotherapy was still mostly experimental at that time. At Harlem Hospital her father had already re-directed the focus of foundation research to investigating anti-cancer chemicals. Dr. Louis Wright worked in the lab and Dr. Jane Wright would perform the patient trials. In 1949, the two began testing a new chemical on human leukemias and cancers of the lymphatic system. Several patients who participated in the trials had some remission. Following Dr. Louis Wright's death in 1952, Dr. Jane Wright was appointed head of the Cancer Research Foundation, at the age of 33.

In 1955, Dr. Wright became an associate professor of surgical research at New York University and director of cancer chemotherapy research at New York University Medical Center and its affiliated Bellevue and University hospitals. In 1964, President Lyndon B. Johnson appointed Dr. Wright to the President's Commission on Heart Disease, Cancer, and Stroke. Based on the Commission's report, a national network of treatment centers was established for these diseases. In 1967, she was named professor of surgery, head of the Cancer Chemotherapy Department, and associate dean at New York Medical College, her alma mater. At a time when African American women physicians numbered only a few hundred in the entire United States, Dr. Wright was the highest ranked African American woman at a created another program to instruct doctors in chemotherapy. In 1971, Dr. Jane Wright became the first woman president of the New York Cancer Society. After a long and fruitful career of cancer research, Dr. Wright retired in 1987. During her forty-year career, Dr. Wright published many research papers on cancer chemotherapy and led delegations of cancer researchers to Africa, China, Eastern Europe, and the Soviet Union.

CHAPTER 12.   NEULASTA TREATMENTS

Neulasta treatments were taken within 24 hours after each chemotherapy treatment.

Neulasta Appts.
1st - 4/4/14
2nd - 4/25/14
3rd - 5/16/14
4th - 6/6/14
5th - 6/27/14
6th - 7/18/14

Neulasta® is a prescription medication used to help reduce the chance of infection due to a low white blood cell count, in people with certain types of cancer (non-myeloid), who receive anti-cancer medicines (chemotherapy) that can cause fever and low blood cell count.[12]

What Can Happen to White Blood Cells During Strong Chemotherapy[13]

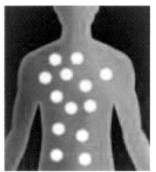

Before chemotherapy:
White blood cells are a key part of your immune system. At natural levels, white blood cells help protect your body against infection.

---

[12] See more at: https://www.neulasta.com/learn-about-neulasta/
[13] See more at: https://www.neulasta.com/low- white-blood-cell-count-cancer/WT.z_co= A&WT.z_in=FN&WT.z_ch=PDS&WT.z_st=&WT.z_mt=&WT.z_pdskw=&WT.z_ag= &WT.z_se=G&WT.srch= 1&WT.z_prm=__&WT.mc_ id=A_FN_PDS_G_____

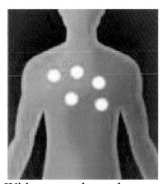

With strong chemotherapy:

Strong chemotherapy can lower the number of infection-fighting white blood cells in your body, which may weaken your immune system and increase your risk for certain types of infection.

The side effects I experienced were mostly weakness in the bones (hands, legs and feet). Today, there is still some weakness in those areas, though not as severe. However, I do need assistance to help with everyday normal household chores such as cooking, cleaning, shopping, opening jars, bottles, etc., lifting packages and other items. I tend to get exhausted quickly when taking on more than I can handle. So, every day I keep the faith, and I continue to pray to God. *Amen.*

It's been almost two months since my diagnosis, but it was the Lord's Day and I wanted to visit Him in church along with everyone else. My husband was definitely down for the cause. It's been a good while since we last been to church, but today was going to be our day.

Getting ready for church, I went into the bathroom and reached for my comb. I then looked into the mirror and began to comb my hair. It was actually starting to fall out — with every stroke of the comb, little by little, tear by tear, my hair was gone. Completely GONE. No way was I going to church — I believe I was in shock for the remainder of the day. And if that wasn't enough to make me lose my mind, I couldn't stop crying. My husband tried almost every tactic in the book to console me. But this challenge had to run its course, I felt. Pity was the last thing I needed at the time. The entire situation was just different for me — I now saw myself as being a "bald-headed woman" as opposed to a woman simply going through chemotherapy. For some reason or another, I just didn't get it. Why? I wish I knew. I guess you have to go through it (or know someone who had) to really understand the ramifications.

It's been six months since I lost my hair and now it was finally growing back and taking shape again. I eventually got the crying down to a sniffle and

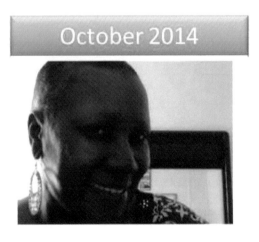

October 2014

began dealing with the new length of my hair. Afterall, I was receiving many compliments from others on the delicacy of my hair. And I did have a nice smile and glow to match it.

In November 2014, I was feeling like a million dollars when I noticed a little more hair growth. While it wasn't exactly extending down my back, it was showing potential growth — and growing out beautifully at that. The texture of it alone felt soft, like baby hair, and I was that baby. It was an opportunity from God to regrow and renurture myself. *Amen.*

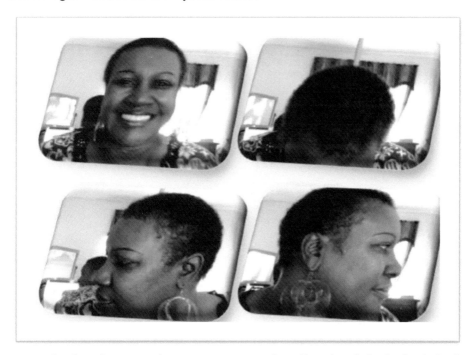

In due time, you learn to mature and realize that it isn't the hair that makes the woman, it's the woman that makes the hair. And then you move on. *Amen.*

Whether you go natural or otherwise (e.g., wig, turban, scarf), it will be your decision. You have to choose what works for you, i.e., what makes you feel better about yourself and work with that. No other person can provide you with these personal revelations but you. No matter what choice you make, life goes on anyway. *Amen.*

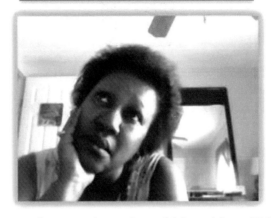

September 2015

Almost a year has gone by and my thick and beautiful hair continues to grow. I'll have to admit that, at the beginning of my hair loss, I wasn't optimistic about its return. But now that an entire year has gone by, its growth has continued to blossom. God does work in mysterious ways. *Amen.*

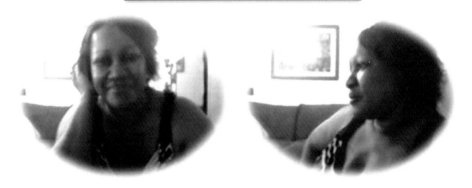

February 20, 2016

Well, it's been a little less than two years since my hair loss and God continues to bless me. My hair is all together and back on track. The texture is still baby soft and delicate and it continues to grow. I haven't actually counted the length in inches but I am counting my blessings. *Amen.*

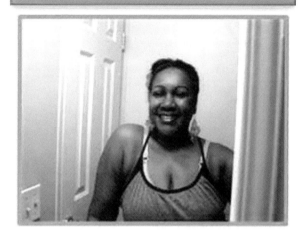

Another four months have passed and the more time goes by, the more beauty grows outside and inside of me. Not only is my hair intact, but so is my soul.

Also, taking vitamins on a regular basis is very essential to my diet. Sometimes there were days that I didn't give myself the necessary nutrients needed, so therefore, I would take my vitamins to substitute for it. And with Nature's Bounty Hair, Skin & Nails, it wasn't an unpleasant taste at all.

14

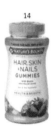

These flavored gummies are delicious and can be taken preferably with your meal — one gummy, twice a day. I saw a big difference in the growth and strength of both my hair and nails as well as the texture of my skin.

---

14 https://www.naturesbounty.com/~/media/naturesbounty/products/products/053545.png?h=360

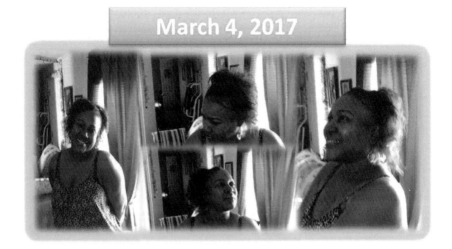

This is me and it's all naturally grown with herbs and spices. My hair is back to its original length and my spirit is astronomical. It's a struggle, but I do manage to take the time and energy to spruce myself up now and then by giving my hair a good home treatment and applying a little makeup to begin my day. But in doing so, I still need my honey, Ed, to support and assist me in my everyday activities. Thank you Lord for bringing such a good man into my life. *Amen.*

I have always defined myself by my features — how I wear my hair, makeup, clothing, etc. Hair loss for me was like a nightmare and when life hits you with a surprise like that, you have no choice but to wake up. Learning and understanding what the true meaning of life is really about is a gift from God. The way I lived prior to my illness will now be conducted in a more positive way — focusing on real matters of life; nurturing and caring for others; keeping God in my life; being forgiving, and then moving on.

Also, having family and friends who support your cause in getting well is always a blessing. Sharing numerous video chats over the Internet involving tips on hairstyles and applying makeup was a major breakthrough for me. Since I was unable to care for myself during my illness, it was a blessing to have my family and friends for support. *Amen.*

CHAPTER 14.   DIET / EXERCISE / MEDITATION / DOCTOR VISITS & MOST OF ALL: 'PRAYER'

My hubby would always say: "IF YOU CAN'T DO A LOT, DO A LITTLE - EVEN A LITTLE MATTERS — IT SHOWS THAT YOU CARE!"

With the love and support of a beautiful husband, how can a girl go wrong? This man has been by my side for the past two decades of my life. We make the best of any situation AND find a solution together as a TEAM.

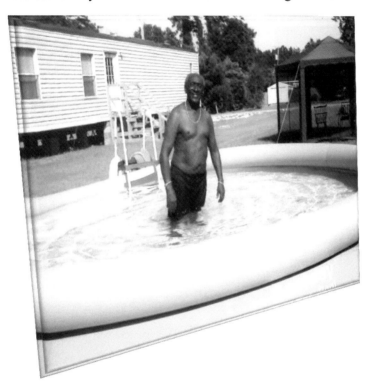

DIET:

Eating healthy was one of our main concerns, but we do like to snack once in a while. During my illness, my favorite drink was chocolate milkshakes. I had to have something sweet because everything else tasted metallic. YULK! You might find yourself temporarily switching to plastic forks, knives and spoons. Metal utensils for me, were definitely not on the menu. Really, you eat just to keep up your strength whether you like it or not. Try to exercise, if possible. Meditation puts you in a completely new place. And always pray to God — in both good and bad times. *Amen.*

As time passes, your taste buds slowly begin to return. Eventually you're back on track. On many occasions, my hubby would prepare healthy and scrumptious meals for us:

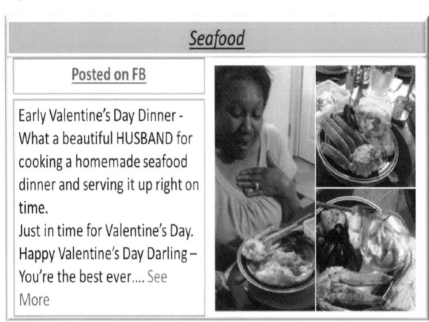

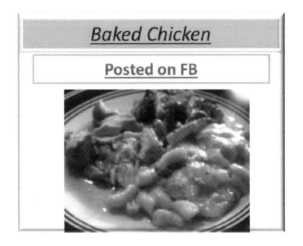

Tuna Salad/Cole Slaw/Strawberries/Apple Sauce

Posted on FB – 6/8/16

OK - TIME FOR A LITTLE HEALTHY BRUNCH!!! AMEN. — eating healthy food.

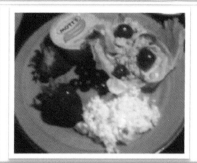

General Tso's Chicken

Posted on FB – 8/12/16

GENERAL TSO'S CHICKEN W/ RICE Ok ya'll, finally HOMEMADE GENERAL TSO'S CHICKEN. Can't believe it — think I'll be doing this from now on. Not only does it look good, it tastes great!!! Nothing like adding in a little something-something like steamed broccoli, yellow/orange/green/red peppers, onions and a little seasoning.

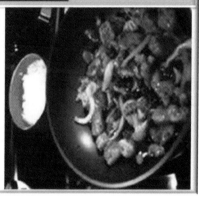

Baked Ziti

Posted on FB – 9/9/16

Nothing like good old homemade baked ziti, collard greens, garlic bread and ziti sauce. God is always good. ALL THE TIME. *AMEN!!!*

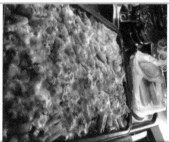

Salisbury Steak
<u>Posted on FB – 9/12/16</u>
Dinner Done Early Tonight: Salisbury Steak in brown gravy, Green Beans, White Rice, Cole Slaw & Homemade Cornbread Muffins — Thank You God for so Many Blessings, *Amen!!!*

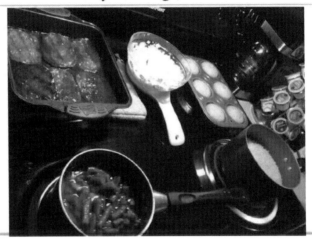

And so many more exciting meals

<u>EXERCISE:</u>

Well, I try to keep my physical strength going, so hopefully, I can get stronger. My 3-lb. weights are accompanying me through it all.

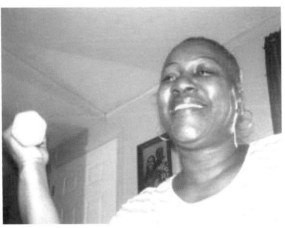

MEDITATION:

Posted on FB – 6/4/16

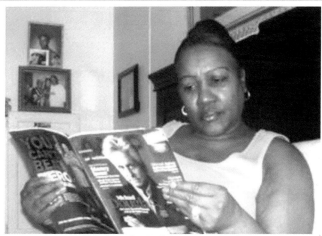

GOOD OLD SATURDAY!
SITTING HERE RESTING MY BONES - TAKING CARE OF ME -
WHEN YOU GET TO BE OVER 50 IT'S TIME FOR MEDITATION AND
AARP. HAVE A BLESSED DAY - *AMEN*!
— 🏀watching X-Men: Apocalypse

Meditation always helps me to recover. Once in a blue moon, I would just go out and walk around the property, gaze at the sun and thank God for it all.

Posted on FB – 7/12/16

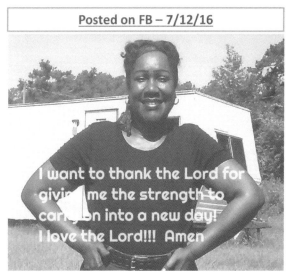

I want to thank the Lord for givin me the strength to carry on into a new day! I love the Lord!!! Amen

It's amazing when someone you love accompanies you to doctor visits, making sure you make each and every appointment. And there my husband was, waiting patiently in the waiting room for my return. I was known to never miss any of my cancer treatment appointments — neulasta treatment, chemotherapy, or any other appointments. I am very proud to say that my husband has always been there to take me where I needed to go. It takes a lot of patience to actually

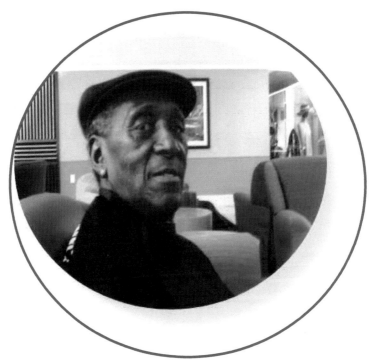

wait for someone in a doctor's office. Depending on test results and other factors, chemotherapy could sometimes take up to six hours to complete. But my husband never failed in keeping me company while waiting for the completion of my treatments. We would play hand-held blackjack, crossword puzzles, Scrabble and Word Finder puzzles to help alleviate some of the pressures of chemotherapy. I love you sweetheart. *God bless you.*

PRAYER:

Practically every day during my illness, my daily prayer consisted of singing this beautiful and emotional gospel song. And where I come from, gospel always soothes the soul:

OH LORD I WANT YOU TO HELP ME[15]

Oh lord I want you to help me
Oh lord I want you to help me
Help me on my journey, help me on my way
Oh lord I want you to help me
While I'm waiting I want you to help me
While I'm waiting I want you to help me
Help me on my journey, help me on my way
Oh lord I want you to help me
Oh lord I want you to help me
Oh lord I want you to help me
Help me on my journey, help me on my way
Oh lord I want you to help me
While I'm singing I want you to help me
While I'm singing I want you to help me
Help me on my journey, help me on my way
Oh lord I want you to help me

Cheryl Pepsii Riley lyrics

---

[15] http://www.lyriczz.com/lyrics/cheryl-pepsii-riley/227841-oh-lord-i-want-you-to-help-me/

170

1.   Ovarian Cancer

NOT COMMON, BUT INCREASING WITH AGE / POSTED ON FRIDAY, JULY 29, 2016 IN WOMEN'S HEALTH[16]

Medically reviewed by Brad Campbell, MD McLeod OB/GYN Associates

A woman's reproductive organs can be affected by five main types of cancer, identified by the location where it started: ovarian, cervical, uterine, vaginal and vulvar.

This article looks at symptoms associated with ovarian cancer. A woman has two ovaries in her pelvis, located on either side of her uterus. They produce the eggs for reproduction as well as some female hormones.

There is no simple, reliable test for ovarian cancer, in the way a Pap test can identify cervical cancer. Making it even more confusing for a woman, many of the symptoms are typical of other non-cancerous problems.

However, if these symptoms are **new** and occur **daily for more than a few weeks,** you should schedule a visit with your gynecologist:

- Pain or swelling in the area below your stomach and between your hip bones.
- Abnormal bleeding or discharge.
- Back pain.
- Feeling full after eating a small amount.
- Gas, bloating, or constipation.
- Sudden or frequent urge to urinate.

---

[16] http://www.mcleodhealth.org/blog/ovarian-cancer-not-common-but-increasing-with-age-1.html

Most or Less at Risk

More Risk

- *Age is one risk factor. About two-thirds of ovarian cancers appear in women 55 or older.*
- *A woman with a sister or mother, who's had ovarian cancer, has increased risk.*
- *Taking an estrogen replacement for 5 years or more. (Women who are treated with a different hormone therapy — progesterone — do not have increased risk.)*

Less Risk

- *Women, who've had multiple children at a young age, have a lower risk.*
- *Women who take birth control pills have lower risk.*

Your Best Defense

"A woman's best defense is a regular exam with her gynecologist to help identify the ovarian cancer," says McLeod Gynecologist Dr. Brad Campbell. "Surgery by a Gynecologic Oncologist is the only cure. These specialists may only be found at academic medical centers. Surgery will probably be followed by chemotherapy. This therapy can be administered at a cancer center close to your home."

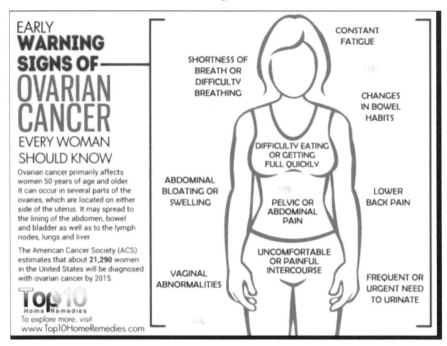

EARLY
**WARNING
SIGNS OF**
OVARIAN
CANCER
EVERY WOMAN
SHOULD KNOW

Ovarian cancer primarily affects
women 50 years of age and older.
It can occur in several parts of the
ovaries, which are located on either
side of the uterus. It may spread to
the lining of the abdomen, bowel
and bladder as well as to the lymph
nodes, lungs and liver.

The American Cancer Society (ACS)
estimates that about **21,290** women
in the United States will be diagnosed
with ovarian cancer by 2015.

Top10
Home Remedies
To explore more, visit
www.Top10HomeRemedies.com

SHORTNESS OF
BREATH OR
DIFFICULTY
BREATHING

CONSTANT
FATIGUE

CHANGES
IN BOWEL
HABITS

DIFFICULTY EATING
OR GETTING
FULL QUICKLY

ABDOMINAL
BLOATING OR
SWELLING

PELVIC OR
ABDOMINAL
PAIN

LOWER
BACK PAIN

UNCOMFORTABLE
OR PAINFUL
INTERCOURSE

VAGINAL
ABNORMALITIES

FREQUENT OR
URGENT NEED
TO URINATE

Baby Powder
& Ovarian Cancer

- Baby powder is widely used
  for a number of tasks,
  including absorbing moisture
  and freshening up

- The product's talcum powder
  base has unfortunately been
  linked to serious health
  problems, including ovarian
  cancer

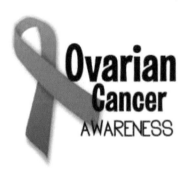

**Ovarian
Cancer**
AWARENESS

---

[17] https://2.bp.blogspot.com/-uIZiPxppt6U/Vx2BumWL_fI/AAAAAAAAB6M/
HYKj7wjtdssTRu7P99dWs1jTmj1iwCwzACLcB/s1600/Screen%2BShot%2B2016-04-
24%2Bat%2B6.48.34%2BPM.png
[18] https://image.slidesharecdn.com/ovariancancerawarenessmonth-150924220329-lva1-
app6891/95/ovarian-cancer-awareness-month-6-638.jpg?cb=1443132402

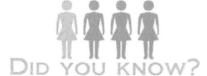

DID YOU KNOW?
1 IN 4 WOMEN DIE DURING
THE FIRST YEAR THEY ARE
DIAGNOSED WITH
OVARIAN CANCER.

THIS IS NOT ACCEPTABLE!!!!
IT'S TIME TO BRING TEAL
TO EVERYONE'S ATTENTION!!

TEAL'S THE DEAL
FOUNDATION

20

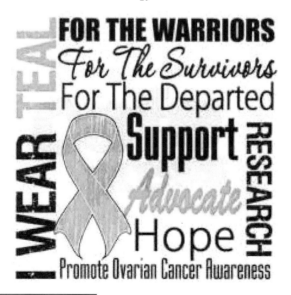

---

[19] https://s-media-cache-ak0.pinimg.com/736x/d3/5b/e1/d35be199e6ed2879
d3ff9919cd31f548.jpg
[20] https://encrypted-tbn1.gstatic.com/images?q=tbn:ANd9GcQvXfpTrxiHxrkp
PtIslcy5gp-WW0qR2svAHc5g4gEx9Z5h6VGt

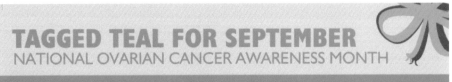

21

Rise up against ovarian cancer™

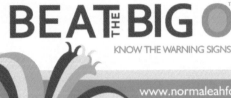

KNOW THE WARNING SIGNS

Bloating that is persistent
Eating less, feeling fuller
Abdominal pain
Trouble with bladder & bowels

www.normaleahfoundation.org and www.cckma-qc.org

2.   **Breast Cancer**

22

Signs & Symptoms

The most common symptom of breast cancer is a new lump or mass. A lump that is painless, hard, and has uneven edges is more likely to be cancer. But some cancers are tender, soft, and rounded or even painful. So it's important to have anything new or unusual checked by a doctor.

Other symptoms of breast cancer include the following:

➢ Swelling of all or part of the breast

➢ Skin irritation or dimpling

➢ Breast pain

➢ Nipple pain or the nipple turning inward

➢ Redness, scaliness , or thickening of the nipple or breast skin

➢ A nipple discharge other than breast milk

Although these symptoms can be caused by things other than breast cancer, it is important to have them checked out by doctor.

---

[21] https://normaleahfoundation.files.wordpress.com/2013/08/2013-tealtag-rgb1.png
[22] https://image.slidesharecdn.com/presentationonbreastcancer-150616225917-lva1-app6891/95/presentation-on-breast-cancer-6-638.jpg?cb=1434495881

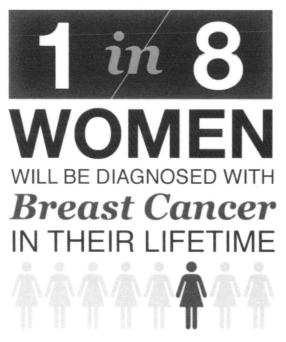

1 in 8 WOMEN
WILL BE DIAGNOSED WITH
Breast Cancer
IN THEIR LIFETIME

October is...
BREAST CANCER AWARENESS
Month
until there is a cure... there is hope

[23] http://s3.amazonaws.com/nbcf-production-assets/attachments/000/000/385/standard_hires/57e514ad84f3780932dff41d5c63ee2c

[24] http://blog.alternativesforseniors.com/wp-content/uploads/2013/10/October-Breast-Cancer.jpg

3.   Lung Cancer

25

SYMPTOMS OF LUNG CANCER

In its early stages, lung cancer normally has no symptoms. When symptoms start to appear, they are usually caused by blocked breathing passages or the spread of cancer further into the lung, surrounding structures, other parts of the body.

Lung cancer symptoms may include:

- Chronic, hacking, raspy coughing, sometimes with blood - streaked mucus.
- Recurring respiratory infections, including bronchitis or pneumonia.
- Increasing shortness of breath, wheezing, persistent chest pain.
- Hoarseness
- Swelling of the neck and face
- Pain and weakness in the shoulder, arm, or hand
- Fatigue, weakness, loss of weight and appetite, intermittent fever, severe headaches, and body pain
- Difficulty swallowing

Medical Observer | Source: WebMD

26

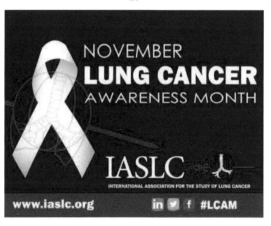

NOVEMBER **LUNG CANCER** AWARENESS MONTH

IASLC
INTERNATIONAL ASSOCIATION FOR THE STUDY OF LUNG CANCER

www.iaslc.org   in f #LCAM

---

25 https://cardsofhope.files.wordpress.com/2014/11/lung-cancer.jpg
26 https://www.iaslc.org/sites/default/files/wysiwyg-assets/lcam16-poster-resized.png

27

Lung Cancer By Age

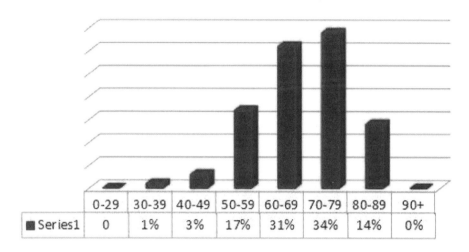

■ Series1	0-29	30-39	40-49	50-59	60-69	70-79	80-89	90+
	0	1%	3%	17%	31%	34%	14%	0%

4.   Uterine Cancer

28

Uterine Cancer—Signs and Symptoms

- Painless vaginal bleeding or spotting is key sign
  - b/c cancer erodes surface tissues
- Pap smear not dependable for detection
- Direct aspiration of cells provides best analysis
- Late signs of malignancy include palpable mass, discomfort or pressure in lower abdomen, bleeding following intercourse

[27] https://www.osfhealthcare.org/media/filer_public_thumbnails/filer_public/fa/7b/fa7ba300-e6c6-4897-ae62-03a3835aa14c/lung_cancer_by_age.jpg__500x301_q85_crop_subsampling-2_upscale.jpg

[28] http://images.slideplayer.com/19/5823467/slides/slide_61.jpg

29

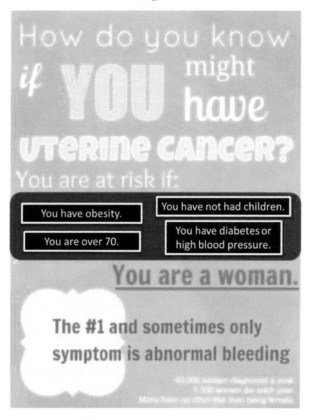

30

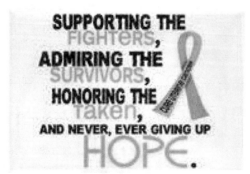

---

[29] https://s-media-cache-ak0.pinimg.com/736x/51/29/41/512941e3460822596bf5b577
930e98f0.jpg

[30] http://i3.cpcache.com/product/617839671/_supporting_admiring_32_uterine
_cancer_shirts_re.jpg?width=225&height=225&Filters=%5B%7B%22name%22%3A%2
2background%22%2C%22value%22%3A%22F2F2F2%22%2C%22sequence%22%3A2
%7D%5D

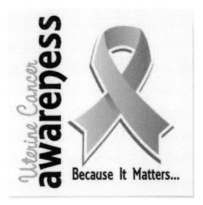

32

Signs of Endometrial / Uterine Cancer

- Abnormal or heavy bleeding
- Difficulty or pain when urinating
- Pain during sexual intercourse
- Some people have no symptoms
- Lack of bleeding
- Watery discharge
- Pain in the pelvic area

Risk Factors

- Overweight
- PCOS
- Early menstruation
- Diabetes
- HRT & High Estrogren
- No pregnancies
- Fibroids & Polyps
- Late menopause

Screening

- Endometrial biopsy
- D&C
- Ultrasound
- MRI & CT Scan

REGULAR CHECKUPS DO NOT SCREEN FOR THIS CANCER!

PLEASE SPEAK UP IF YOU ARE EXPERIENCING ANY OF THESE SYMPTOMS!

---

[31] https://rlv.zcache.com/uterine_cancer_awareness_5_poster-r3020435222b949 b9b74ef9337a0e9e35_wad_8byvr_324.jpg

[32] https://s-media-cache-ak0.pinimg.com/736x/b7/02/12/b70212a998be3ccc bf3f4d9391151c07.jpg

5. Colon Cancer

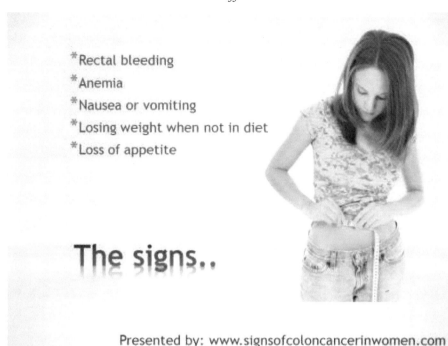

33

*Rectal bleeding
*Anemia
*Nausea or vomiting
*Losing weight when not in diet
*Loss of appetite

The signs..

Presented by: www.signsofcoloncancerinwomen.com

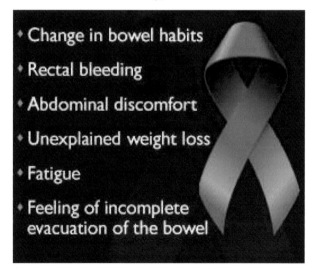

* Change in bowel habits
* Rectal bleeding
* Abdominal discomfort
* Unexplained weight loss
* Fatigue
* Feeling of incomplete evacuation of the bowel

---

[33] https://i.ytimg.com/vi/N2WkSgm076w/maxresdefault.jpg
[34] http://www.buzzle.com/img/articleImages/357008-9428-47.jpg

COLON CANCER OFTEN HAS NO OBVIOUS SIGNS OR SYMPTOMS.

FACT! Regular screening is the key to early detection because, in many cases, by the time symptoms appear, the cancer may have already advanced to a later stage.

BeSeenGetScreened.com

36

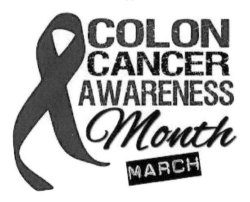

35 https://s-media-cache-ak0.pinimg.com/236x/79/4a/02/794a02a6ee96a461404
f0f501057c70b.jpg
36 http://elpasoheraldpost.com/wp-content/uploads/2016/03/march_colon
_cancer_awareness.jpg

6.   Liver Cancer

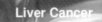

Liver Cancer

❖ Liver cancer is a cancer which originates in the liver

❖ There are 4 main types
- Hepatocellular carcinoma (HCC)
- Cholangiocarcinoma
- Angiosarcoma
- Hepatoblastoma

❖ The major types is Hepatocellular carcinoma (HCC)

Sign & Symptom

❖ **Sign and symptom of liver cancer is no specific**
- abdominal mass
- abdominal pain
- emesis
- anemia
- back pain
- jaundice
- itching
- weight loss
- Fever

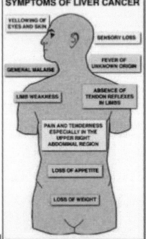

SYMPTOMS OF LIVER CANCER

---

[37] https://image.slidesharecdn.com/assignment2-livercancerdiagnosticsgroup3-150921152732-lva1-app6891/95/liver-cancer-diagnostics-and-future-trends-3-638.jpg?cb=1442849340
[38] http://image.slidesharecdn.com/assignment2-livercancerdiagnosticsgroup3-150921152732-lva1-app6891/95/liver-cancer-diagnostics-and-future-trends-4-638.jpg?cb=1442849340

Symptoms

Most people don't have signs and symptoms in the early stages of primary liver cancer. When signs and symptoms do appear, they may include:

- Losing weight without trying

- Loss of appetite

- Upper abdominal pain

- Nausea and vomiting

- General weakness and fatigue

- An enlarged liver

- Abdominal swelling

- Yellow discoloration of your skin and the whites of your eyes

- White, chalky stools

40

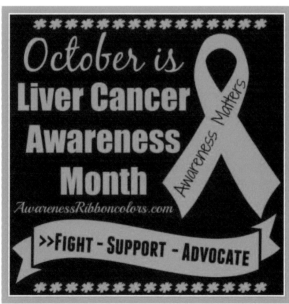

---

[39] https://image.slidesharecdn.com/liverproblems-130604104729-phpapp01/95/liver-problems-4-638.jpg?cb=1370342913
[40] https://s-media-cache-ak0.pinimg.com/originals/3a/99/41/3a99410ed39711290dc0b9f4b190d793.jpg

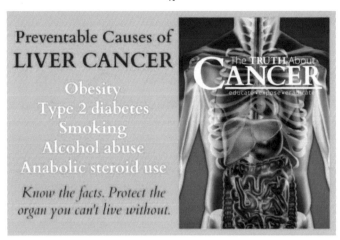

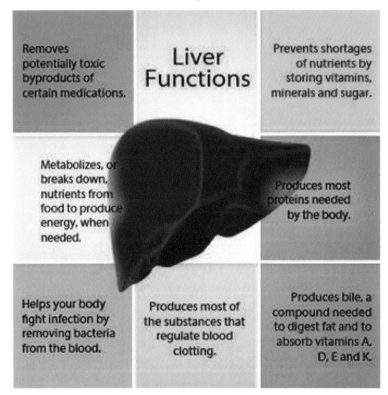

---

[41] https://s3.amazonaws.com/ttac-com/wp-content/uploads/TTAC-Liver-Cancer-Graphic.jpg

[42] https://s-media-cache-ak0.pinimg.com/originals/b8/a9/71/b8a97150c1bf6d10ea9715d4b8a5ca3b.jpg

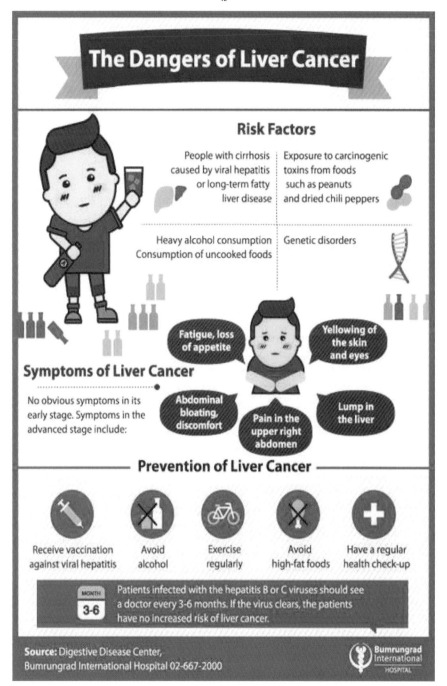

[43] https://www.bumrungrad.com/getattachment/b845216f-5b06-40aa-832f-f03fc6431490/
529-749-liver-cancer-infographic.jpg;;.aspx

7.   Autism

44

For in-depth information and safety tips, please visit NAA's Autism Safety site[45].

Drowning is among the leading causes of death of individuals with autism. Please click here for a list of YMCA locations[46] that offer special needs swimming lessons, and be sure that your child's last lesson is with clothes and shoes on.

Overall Mortality
- In 2008, Danish researchers found that the mortality risk among the autism population is twice as high as the general population
- In 2001, a California research team found elevated deaths in autism and attributed it to several causes, including seizures and accidents such as suffocation and drowning

Wandering/Elopement
- Roughly half, or 48%, of children with an ASD attempt to elope from a safe environment, a rate nearly four times higher than their unaffected siblings
- In 2009, 2010, and 2011, accidental drowning accounted for 91% total U.S. deaths reported in children with an ASD ages 14 and younger subsequent to wandering/elopement.
- More than one third of ASD children who wander/elope are never or rarely able to communicate their name, address, or phone number
- Two in three parents of elopers reported their missing children had a "close call" with a traffic injury
- 32% of parents reported a "close call" with a possible drowning
- Wandering was ranked among the most stressful ASD behaviors by 58% of parents of elopers
- 62% of families of children who elope were prevented from attending/enjoying activities outside the home due to fear of wandering
- 40% of parents had suffered sleep disruption due to fear of elopement
- Children with ASD are eight times more likely to elope between the ages of 7 and 10 than their typically-developing siblings
- Half of families with elopers report they had never received advice or guidance about elopement from a professional
- Only 19% had received such support from a psychologist or mental health professional
- Only 14% had received guidance from their pediatrician or another physician

Source: Interactive Autism Network Research Report: Elopement and Wandering

(2011)

Source: National Autism Association, Lethal Outcomes in ASD Wandering (2012)

---

[44] For more information go to: http://nationalautismassociation.org/resources/ autism-safety-facts/
[45] For more information go to: http://www.autismsafety.org/
[46] For list of YMCA locations go to: http://nationalautismassociation.org/resources/ autism-safety-facts/swimming-instructions/

The National Center for Missing and Exploited Children has recently published an important document for first responders and search and rescue personnel for cases involving an individual with special needs. Please visit this link, print and share this document[47] with your local police, sheriff and fire departments.

Restraint/Seclusion
- It's estimated that over the last five years, more than 20 students, many with disabilities, have died due to seclusion and restraints being used in schools.
- A 2009 Government Accountability Office (GAO) investigation reported that thousands of students have been physically injured and emotionally traumatized as the result of restraint and seclusion
- Currently there is no federal law that prohibits the use of restraints that restrict breathing, and locked seclusion, in public and private schools.
- Dangers include: Death by asphyxiation; Bodily injury; Post Traumatic Stress Disorder; Heart, gastrointestinal and pulmonary complications; Decreased appetite and malnutrition; Dehydration; Urinary tract infections; Incontinence; Agitation; Depression/withdrawal; Loss of dignity; Sleeping problems; Humiliation; Anxiety; Increased phobias; Increased aggression, including SIB (self-injurious behavior)

Source: United States Government Accountability Office, Selected Cases of Death and Abuse at Public and Private Schools and Treatment Center (2009)

Bullying
- 65% of parents reported that their children with Asperger's syndrome had been victimized by peers in some way within the past year
- 47% reported that their children had been hit by peers or siblings
- 50% reported them to be scared by their peers
- 9% were attacked by a gang and hurt in the private parts
- 12% indicated their child had never been invited to a birthday party
- 6% were almost always picked last for teams
- 3% ate alone at lunch every day

Source: Issues in Comprehensive Pediatric Nursing (2009)

Sexual Abuse
- According to the Centers for Disease Control and Prevention (CDC), approximately 1 in 6 boys and 1 in 4 girls suffer from sexual abuse before the age of 18.
- Additionally, the U.S. Department of Justice's National Crime Victimization Survey, the country's largest and most reliable crime study, reports that every two minutes a person is sexually victimized in the United States—and the numbers for individuals with disabilities are even higher.
- A study done in Nebraska of 55,000 children showed a child with any type of intellectual disability was four times more likely to be sexually abused than a child without disabilities (Sullivan & Knutson, 2000). While no specific numbers exist for individuals with autism, research suggests that this population is extremely vulnerable.

---

[47] For more information go to: http://www.missingkids.com/en_US/publications/ SpecialNeeds_Addendum.pdf

NAA has set up 3 specific Autism & Safety groups on Facebook. Join these pages for relevant news, action alerts and updates pertaining to these topics.

48   49   50

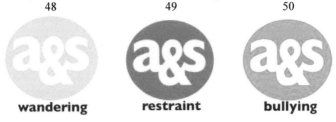

wandering   restraint   bullying

51

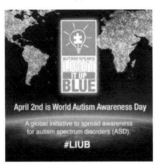

52

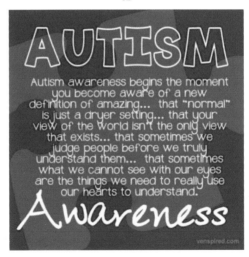

---

[48] For information go to: https://www.facebook.com/AutismWandering
[49] For information go to: https://www.facebook.com/AutismRestraint
[50] For information go to: https://www.facebook.com/AutismBullying
[51] https://www.autismspeaks.org/news/news-item/celebrities-who-went-blue-world-autism-awareness-day
[52] https://nataliehanson.com/2014/04/02/autism-awareness-2014/

8.   Thyroid Disease

53

SIGNS & SYMPTOMS

- Most thyroid nodules don't cause signs or symptoms.
- Occasionally some may become so large that they can feel or even see the swelling at the base of the neck, especially when shaving or putting on makeup.
- Men sometimes become aware of a nodule because their shirt collars suddenly feel too tight.
- Some nodules produce too much thyroxine, a hormone secreted by the thyroid gland.

54

What are the symptoms of thyroid disease?

Table 1

Symptoms of Thyroid Disease			
Hyperthyroidism (Overactive) % Cases		Hyperthyroidism (Underactive) % Cases	
Rapid heart rate	100	Weakness	99
Goiter	100	Dry or course skin	97
Nervousness	99	Fatigue	91
Tremor	97	Slow speech	91
Increased swelling	91	Swelling of eyelids	90
Heart intolerance	89	Cold intolerance	89
Palpitation	89	Thick tongue	82
Fatigue	88	Slow movements	80
Weight loss	85	Swelling of face	79
Trouble breathing or shortage of breath	66	Memory impairment	75
Weakness	70	Constipation	61
Increased appetite	65	Weight gain	59
Eye complaints	40	Hair loss	57
Log swelling	55	Trouble breathing or shortage of breath	35
Increased bowel habit	33	Ankle swelling	55
Poor appetite	9	Menstrual problems	32
Constipation	4	Goiter	30
Weight gain	2	Slowed heart rate	10

---

[53] https://image.slidesharecdn.com/thyroiddysfunction-edited-100202000028-phpapp02/95/thyroid-dysfunctionppt-10-728.jpg?cb=1273476918
[54] http://www.familyhealthonline.ca/FHsfwy/fho/familymedicine/FM_thyroid_FHc05.asp

The most common symptoms and signs associated with thyroid disease are compared in Table 1. Many of these are non-specific, which means they occur in a variety of different diseases. This can make it difficult for doctors to arrive at a quick diagnosis without the benefit of several blood tests. However, routine testing in adults without signs or symptoms suggestive of thyroid disease should not be done.

In extreme cases, abnormal thyroid hormone levels can have serious results. If the level gets very low a condition called myxedema can occur. In its worst form, it can cause coma and death. Extremely high levels of thyroid hormone can cause seizures and mental illness (thyroid storm). Thankfully, these extremes are very rare these days.

[55]

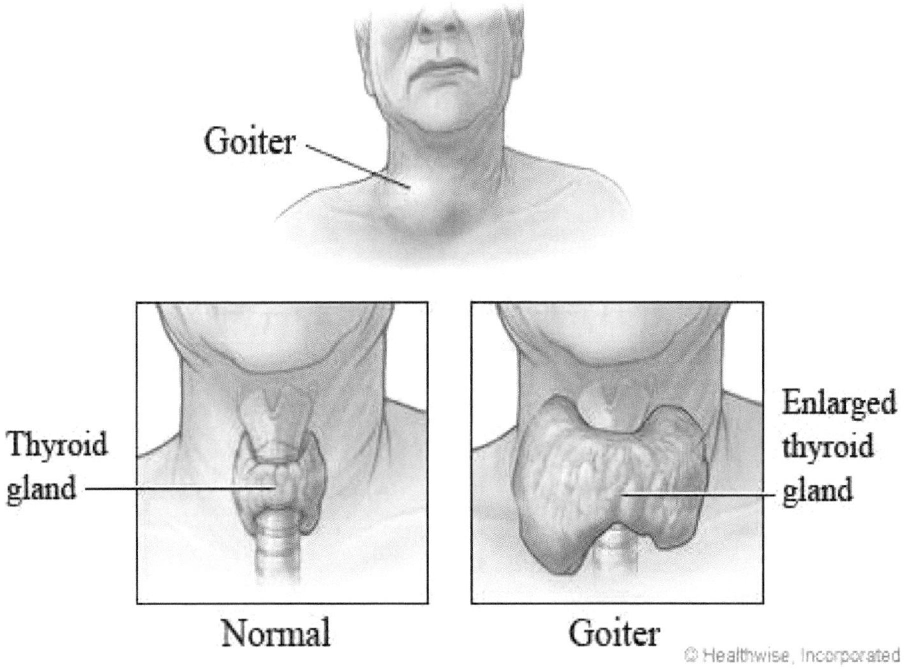

© Healthwise, Incorporated

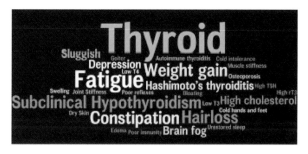

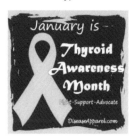

9. Epilepsy & Seizures

Classifying Seizures

Focal (previously 'partial') seizure – initial activation of only part of one cerebral hemisphere occurs. (although may generalize*)

Generalized seizure – discharge from both cerebral hemispheres occurs. Loss of consciousness may occur.

- Seizure types:

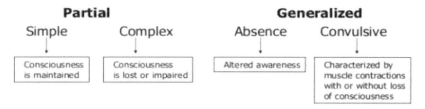

---

56 https://encrypted-tbn0.gstatic.com/images?q=tbn:ANd9GcSAwPMKorddBFvj6
MmsM3ozbYX1cZQBDZt_u3nbsuTrwa4ZaRDo

57 https://66.media.tumblr.com/f024f2cb7782bbf17e6e5e87168577fd/tumblr_
nheyzgZuUs1r6iga9o1_500.png

58 http://image.slidesharecdn.com/typesofseizure-130818163352-phpapp01/95/types-of-
seizure-6-638.jpg?cb=1376843698

EPILEPSY & SEIZURES:

Know What To Do!

DO

- Cushion the person's head and remove dangerous obstacles.
- Turn the person on his side.
- Time the seizure.
- Loosen tight clothing, especially ties and collars.

DON'T

- Hold the person down.
- Put anything in the person's mouth.
- Panic. Stay calm, and call 911 if necessary.

lauren's
HOPE

WWW.LAURENSHOPE.COM

Seizure Triggers or Precipitants

- A student's environment or activities may need to be modified to reduce exposure to situations that trigger seizures.
- A school safety evaluation can help determine any changes that need to be made.
- Consider flashing lights in MOVIES, TELEVISION and COMPUTERS, all of which can be seizure triggers.
- In many cases there is no identifiable trigger or precipitating factor.

EPILEPSY
FOUNDATION

24

---

[59] https://www.consumerhealthdigest.com/health-awareness/national-epilepsy-awareness-month.html

[60] www.slideshare.net/dembry-wcps/seizures-13928348

November Is Epilepsy Awareness Month

Epilepsy Is A Neurological Condition That Produces Brief Disturbances In The Normal Electrical Functions Of The Brain That Can Cause People To Have Seisures. Epilepsy Is Non-Discriminatory And Effects More Than 3 Million People In The United States.

Here In Connecticut Approximately 60,000 People Have Epilepsy. 1 In 10 People Will Have Some Type Of Seisure.Research To Find A Cure Is Ongoing.

10. High Blood Pressure

62

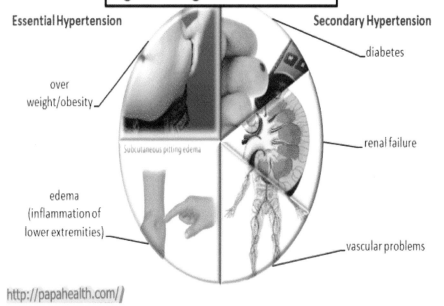

61 https://i.ytimg.com/vi/BUleb8FvVyQ/maxresdefault.jpg
62 https://userscontent2.emaze.com/images/3be99f6a-95e7-44e6-baa0-54c1a835ff70/05054080117a4773ce586aa018f5ec01.gif

63

ARE YOU A LIKELY CANDIDATE FOR HIGH BLOOD PRESSURE?

If so, it will be even more important for you to manage your lifestyle with heart-healthier habits. Science has identified several factors that can increase your risk of developing high blood pressure (HBP) and thus your risk for heart attack, heart disease and stroke.

Risks among certain groups:

- African-Americans — If you're African American, there's a good chance that you or a relative has HBP.

- Women — Starting at age 65, women are more likely to have high blood pressure than men.

- Children — While HBP is most common in adults, children can develop it too.

64

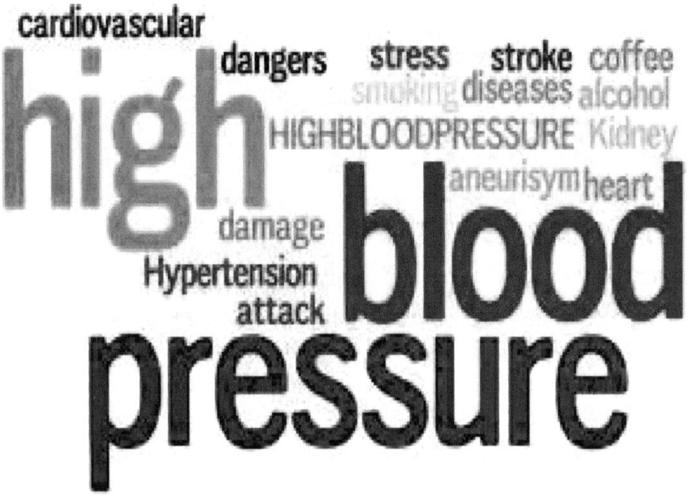

---

[63] See more http://www.heart.org/HEARTORG/Conditions/HighBloodPressure/
UnderstandYourRiskforHighBloodPress/Understand-Your-Risk-for-High-Blood-
Pressure_UCM_002052_Article.jsp
[64] http://med-x.in/wp-content/uploads/2016/01/HTNBP.jpg

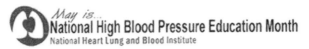

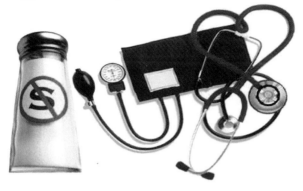

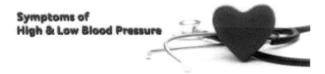

Common symptoms of high blood pressure
1. Breathlessness
2. Headache
3. Bleeding from the nose
4. Fatigue and Sleepiness
5. Confusion
6. Vomiting
7. Profuse sweating and
8. Blurred vision

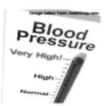

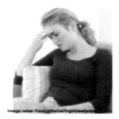

Common symptoms of low blood pressure:
1. Dizziness and light-heartedness
2. Pain in the chest
3. Black or maroon coloured stools
4. Irregular heart beat
5. Head ache
6. Back pain or Stiff neck
7. Consistent high fever
8. Burning sensation in the urine

If you do not have the above symptoms, it does not mean that you have no high or low blood pressure at all. Remember that the most common is that "It Has No Symptom". The best way to maintain your health and is to have your blood pressure checked at frequent intervals.

---

65 https://s-media-cache-ak0.pinimg.com/originals/45/c7/18/45c718b462fc77
4793a3fcc650e92e38.jpg
66 http://www.healthnavigator.org.nz/media/1002/blood-pressure-hf-2015.jpg

11. Stroke

67

MAY IS STROKE AWARENESS MONTH

STOP Stroke • Act F.A.S.T. • Spread HOPE

68

Signs & Symptoms of a Stroke

Five Warning Signs:

1. **Sudden severe headache**
For no apparent reason

2. **Sudden weakness**
Numbness and/or tingling in
the face, arm or leg

3. **Sudden dizziness**
Unsteadiness or sudden falls,
especially with any of the other
warning signs

4. **Sudden vision trouble**
Sudden loss of vision (sight),
particularly in one eye,
or double vision

5. **Sudden speech trouble**
Temporary loss of speech or
trouble understanding speech

**If you notice one or more
of these signs, don't wait... CALL 911**

A stroke increases your risk of having another stroke.

---

[67] http://www.healingsinmotion.org/wp-content/uploads/2013/05/stroke-awareness.jpg
[68] https://s-media-cache-ak0.pinimg.com/originals/cd/36/66/cd36665b6fd159704
54e16abdc73d725.jpg

12.   Heart Attack

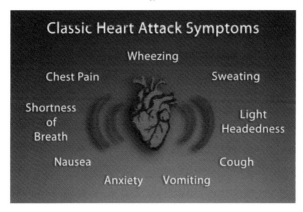

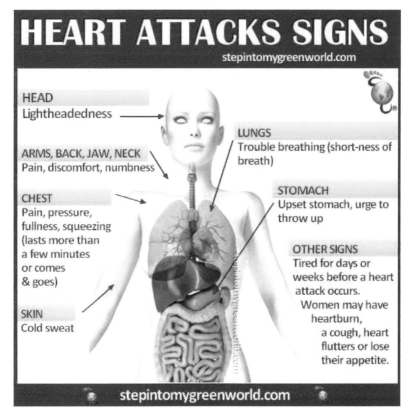

---

[69] http://elitemensguide.com/assets/Signs-of-Heart-Attack.png
[70] https://s-media-cache-ak0.pinimg.com/originals/7a/e6/55/7ae6557ea87efb252
cfecd74f2c140e7.png

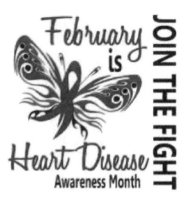

13. Gout

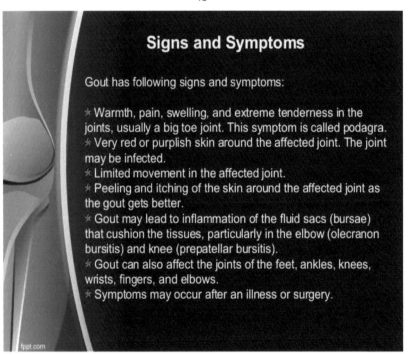

[71] https://rlv.zcache.ca/heart_disease_awareness_month_butterfly_3_1_postcard-ra59da91c3f9e4029b03f70118b50c56b_vgbaq_8byvr_324.jpg
[72] https://image.slidesharecdn.com/getyourgoutproblemsolvedatspecialized arthritisandmedicalclinicsinsingapore-150421022908-conversion-gate02/95/get-your-gout-problem-solved-at-specialized-arthritis-and-medical-clinics-in-singapore-3-638.jpg?cb=1429583404

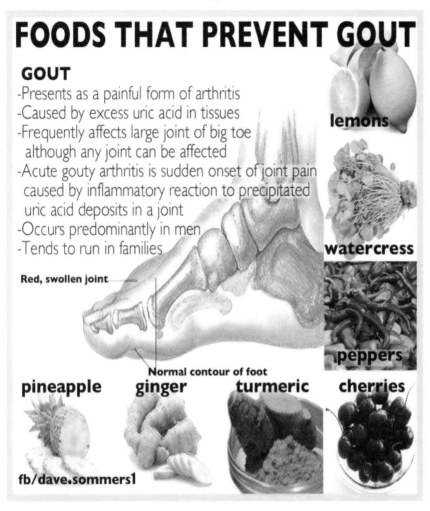

FOODS THAT PREVENT GOUT

GOUT

-Presents as a painful form of arthritis
-Caused by excess uric acid in tissues
-Frequently affects large joint of big toe
  although any joint can be affected
-Acute gouty arthritis is sudden onset of joint pain
  caused by inflammatory reaction to precipitated
  uric acid deposits in a joint
-Occurs predominantly in men
-Tends to run in families

lemons

watercress

peppers

Red, swollen joint

Normal contour of foot

pineapple **ginger** **turmeric** **cherries**

fb/dave.sommers1

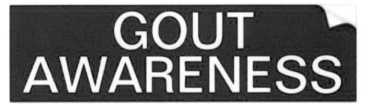

GOUT AWARENESS

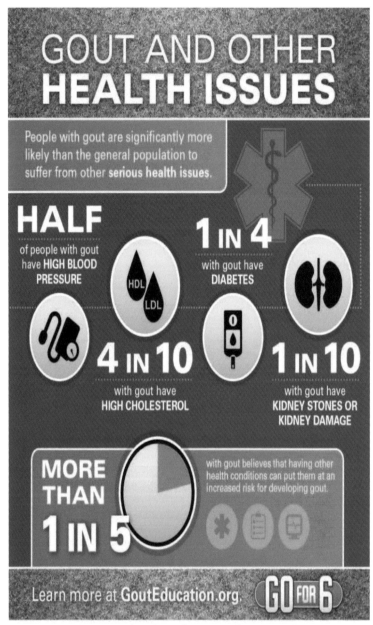

Online survey of American adults and gout sufferers conducted in
April 2016 on behalf of the Gout & Uric Acid Education Society.

[75] http://gouteducation.org/wp-content/uploads/2016/05/GUAES-Infographic_Other-Health-Issues_FINAL.jpg

14. Gangrene

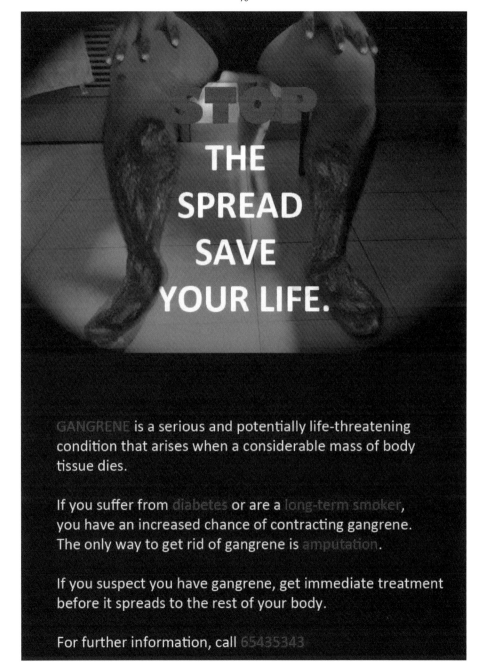

GANGRENE is a serious and potentially life-threatening condition that arises when a considerable mass of body tissue dies.

If you suffer from diabetes or are a long-term smoker, you have an increased chance of contracting gangrene. The only way to get rid of gangrene is amputation.

If you suspect you have gangrene, get immediate treatment before it spreads to the rest of your body.

For further information, call 65435343

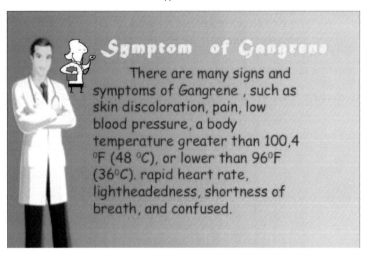

SEPTEMBER
Peripheral Arterial Disease (PAD) Awareness Month

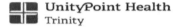 UnityPoint Health
Trinity

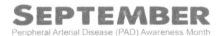

PAD develops when arteries become clogged with plaque and fatty deposits that limit blood flow to legs.

PAD affects 8 TO 12 MILLION people in the United States

People with PAD have 4-5 times GREATER RISK for heart attack or stroke

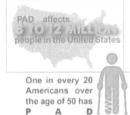

One in every THREE people over the age of 50 with diabetes is likely to have PAD

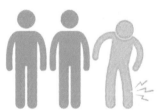

One in every 20 Americans over the age of 50 has PAD

PAD often goes UNDERDIAGNOSED by healthcare professionals

Left untreated, PAD can lead to GANGRENE and AMPUTATION

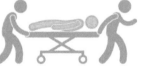

Timely detection and treatment of PAD can improve patient's QUALITY OF LIFE; reduce risk of heart attack, stroke, leg amputation and even death

65% of patients undergoing limb amputation in the US did not have an ABI (ankle brachial index) documented

· American Heart Association (www.heart.org) · US Department of Health and Human Services. National Institutes of Health. National Heart, Lung, and Blood Institute · www.amputee-coalition.org/healthcare-providers/limb-loss-statistics/index.html Hirsch AT. Circulation 2007:116:2086-2094 Endovascular Today March 2006

To refer a patient, contact us at 1-800-379-HEAL
Bettendorf, IA 563-742-5100 | Moline, IL 309-779-5395

Healogics

---

[77] https://image.slidesharecdn.com/kelompok3-140408053139-phpapp 01/95/gangrene-3-638.jpg?cb=1396935203
[78] https://media.licdn.com/mpr/mpr/shrinknp_800_800/AAEAAQAAAAAAAIU AAAAJGU1OWNlNWU2LWEwZDctNDQ2My1hZjk0LTUzMzAxYzZhOTcwOQ.jpg

79

Consequences of Enlarged Prostate:

Symptoms of enlarget prostate	When do they occur	How to manage
Sleep disorders	Due to right "washroom visits"	Try to reduce prime symptoms
Psychological disorders: - Irritability - Stressed	Because of the non-managet enlarget prostatesymptoms	Chamommile tea, or other tranquilizant drugs(with your doctor prescription)
General: - Weakness - Fatigue	Especially at the last unmanaged stage	After managing the symptoms, herbs, vitamins and minerals boost

www.prostate-treatment-options.com

80

6 Natural Remedies for Enlarged Prostate

The Prostate Grows

The prostate is a walnut-shaped gland that wraps around the urethra (the tube that outflows urine). It's part of a man's reproductive system. One of its main jobs is to add fluid (called semen) to sperm. Although the gland starts out small, it tends to enlarge as a man ages. An excessively enlarged prostate results in a disease known as benign prostatic hyperplasia (BPH). Eventually, an enlarged prostate can clamp down on the urethra, restricting the flow of urine from the bladder. This leads to problems such as frequent urination, difficulty in voiding, urinary leakage, and urinary tract infections.

---

[79] http://www.prostate-treatment-options.com/images/consequenses-of-enlarget-prostate.jpg
[80] https://image.slidesharecdn.com/6naturalremediesforenlargedprostate-160320163551/95/6-natural-remedies-for-enlarged-prostate-1-638.jpg?cb=1458491761

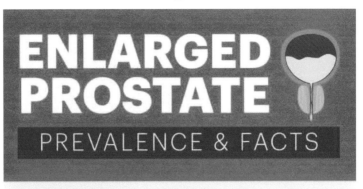

ENLARGED PROSTATE
PREVALENCE & FACTS

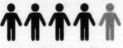

Enlarged prostate affects

1 in 5 men

between the ages of 50
and 60, and it's even more
common in older men

BPH is the most common
noncancerous form of cell
growth in men

About 1/3 of men with an
enlarged prostate have lower
urinary tract symptoms that
can interfere with their
quality of life

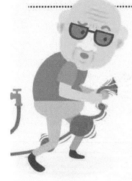

Men with enlarged prostate may suddenly have
difficulty urinating, or they cannot urinate at all,
because they have acute urinary retention

Enlargement of the prostate gland develops as a
strictly age-related phenomenon in nearly all men,
starting at approximately 40 years of age

Prevalence of BPH is approximately:

10%

for men in
their 30s

20%

for men in
their 40s

50%-60%

for men in
their 60s

80%-90%

for men in their
70s and 80s

Dr. Axe
FOOD IS MEDICINE

---

81 https://draxe.com/wp-content/uploads/2016/11/ProstateGraphic.jpg

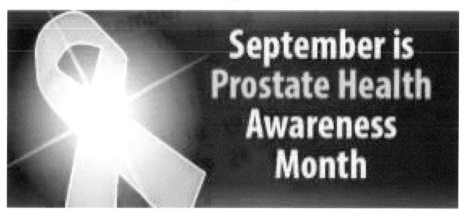

16.   Prostate Cancer

83

84

What Men Need to Know

September is Prostate Cancer Awareness Month

About 233,000 new cases of prostate cancer will be diagnosed.

About 29,480 men will die of prostate cancer.

1 man out of 7 will be diagnosed with prostate cancer during his lifetime.

RISK FACTORS

AGE
The older a man is, the greater his risk for getting prostate cancer.

FAMILY HISTORY
Certain genes that you inherited may affect your prostate cancer risk. A man with a father, brother or son who has had prostate cancer is two to three times more likely to develop the disease himself.

RACE
Prostate cancer occurs more often in African-American men than in white men.

SIGNS & SYMPTOMS

Different people have different symptoms for prostate cancer. Some men do not have symptoms at all.

Some symptoms of prostate cancer are:

- Difficulty starting urination
- Weak or interrupted flow of urine
- Frequent urination, especially at night
- Difficulty emptying the bladder completely
- Pain or burning during urination
- Blood in the urine or semen
- Pain in the back, hips, or pelvis that doesn't go away

SCREENINGS

DIGITAL RECTAL EXAM (DRE)
A doctor or nurse inserts a gloved, lubricated finger into the rectum to estimate the size of the prostate and feel for lumps or other abnormalities.

PROSTATE SPECIFIC ANTIGEN (PSA) TEST
Measures the level of PSA in the blood. PSA is a substance made by the prostate. The levels of PSA in the blood can be higher in men who have prostate cancer. The PSA level may also be elevated in other conditions that affect the prostate.

HARRIS**HEALTH** SYSTEM

84 https://harrishealth.files.wordpress.com/2014/09/infographic-harris-health-prostate.jpg?w=551&h=1376

17.   **Shingles**

85

What causes Shingles?

Most people have chickenpox in childhood, but after the illness has gone, the virus remains dormant (inactive) in the nervous system. The immune system keeps the virus in check, but later in life it can be reactivated and cause shingles.

It is not known exactly why the shingles virus is reactivated at a later stage in life, but most cases are thought to be caused by having lowered immunity (protection against infections and diseases).

This may be the result of:

- being older
- being stressed
- taking medication that weakens your immune system
- a condition that affects your immune system, such as HIV or AIDS

86

Who's at special risk?

Some children and adults are at special risk of serious problems if they catch chickenpox. They include:

- pregnant women
- new-born babies
- people with a weakened immune system

These people should seek medical advice as soon as they are exposed to the chickenpox virus or they develop chickenpox symptoms.

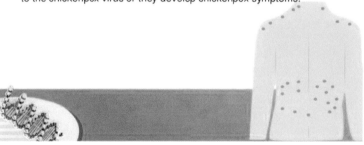

---

85 https://image.slidesharecdn.com/chickenpoxandshinglesprescompleted-151118041329-lva1-app6891/95/the-cause-symptoms-and-treatments-for-chickenpox-and-shingles-9-638.jpg?cb=1447820755

86 https://image.slidesharecdn.com/chickenpoxandshinglesprescompleted-151118041329-lva1-app6891/95/the-cause-symptoms-and-treatments-for-chickenpox-and-shingles-5-638.jpg?cb=1447820755

87

MODE OF TRANSMISSION

- Chickenpox is transmitted from **person to person.**

- by directly **touching the blisters, saliva or mucus of an infected person.**

- The virus can also be **transmitted through the air by coughing and sneezing.**

- Chickenpox can be **spread indirectly by touching contaminated items freshly soiled, such as clothing, from an infected person.**

- Direct contact with the blisters of a person with shingles can cause chickenpox in a person who has never had chickenpox and has not been vaccinated.

- Blisters that are dry and crusted are no longer able to spread chickenpox.

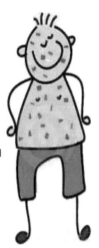

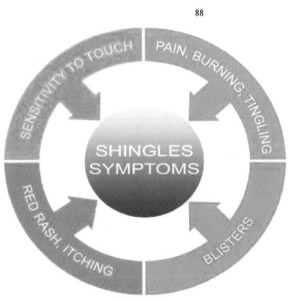

---

[87] https://image.slidesharecdn.com/presentation1-131103053443-phpapp 02/95/varicella-zoster-5-638.jpg?cb=1404980926

[88] https://www.consumerhealthdigest.com/wp-content/uploads/2015/03/symptoms-of-shingles.jpg

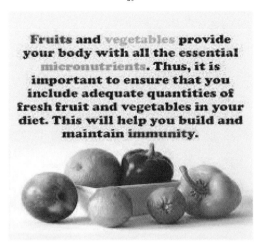

Fruits and vegetables **provide your body with all the essential** micronutrients. **Thus, it is important to ensure that you include adequate quantities of fresh fruit and vegetables in your diet. This will help you build and maintain immunity.**

18. Lupus

90

Common Signs & Symptoms of Lupus

- Painful or swollen joints and muscle pain
- Unexplained fever
- Red rashes, most commonly on the face
- Chest pain upon deep breathing
- Unusual loss of hair
- Raynaud's phenomenon
- Sensitivity to the sun
- Edema in legs or around eyes
- Mouth ulcers
- Swollen glands
- Extreme fatigue

U.S. Department of Health and Human Services. National Institutes of Health. National Institute of Arthritis and Musculoskeletal and Skin Diseases. NIH Publication No. 03-4178. August 2003.

---

[89] https://encrypted-tbn1.gstatic.com/images?q=tbn:ANd9GcRMFoAWxgzqU2L PxoS_EIIzB7Dq44fbFhaLpacRwdo9auVgOkZz0Q

[90] https://image.slidesharecdn.com/dr-dan-wallace-presents-at-lupus-las-annual-patient-education-conference-120041842044671-3/95/dr-dan-wallace-presents-new-therapies-for-lupus-and-clinical-trials-at-lupus-las-annual-patient-education-conference-5-728.jpg?cb=1200389620

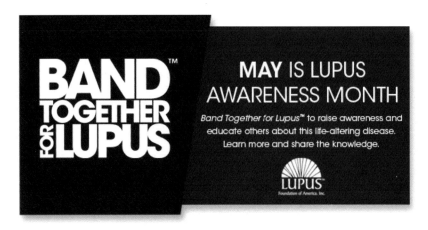

Warning Signs of Lupus

When lupus first sets in, symptoms such as fatigue and pain are often non-specific. They can be signs of so many other health problems, which can make diagnosis hard. The most common complaint people have is fatigue that is so severe it stops them from being able to function normally. This fatigue is often related to fibromyalgia. Fever, muscle and joint pain are also quite common.

Muscle & Joint Pain
95% of people with lupus experience muscle and joint pain.

Fever Greater Than 100° F
90% of people with lupus get a fever of more than 100 degrees Fahrenheit (38 degrees Celsius).

Prolonged or Extreme Fatigue
81% of people with lupus suffer from prolonged or extreme fatigue.

Anemia
71% of people with lupus simultaneously suffer from anemia.

---

[91] https://s-media-cache-ak0.pinimg.com/originals/74/cf/3e/74cf3ea7187347bcd894226b22f6852e.jpg

[92] https://image.slidesharecdn.com/lupusceu-120926211438-phpapp02/95/lupus-4-728.jpg?cb=1348694228

19.   Arthritis

93

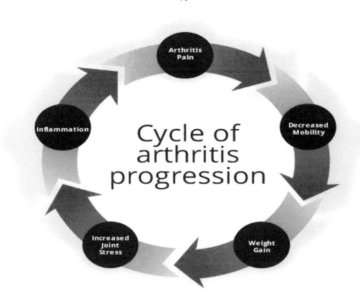

94

Arthritis :

Arthritis is nothing but disorders of joint that involves inflammation of one or more joints. There are various types of arthritis like osteoarthritis or degenerative arthritis, rheumatoid arthritis, rheumatic arthritis, gout or pseudo arthritis, psoriatic arthritis, stills disease, septic arthritis, reactive arthritis, arthritis from SLE origin etc. Among them most common for m of arthritis are osteoarthritis and rheumatoid arthritis. In any form of arthritis the most common symptoms are restriction of movement with stiffness of joint.

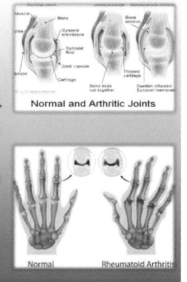

---

93 http://www.westmountanimalclinic.com/wp-content/uploads/2014/03/arthritis-cycle.png

94 https://image.slidesharecdn.com/nowarthritiscaneasilycurableinhomeopathy treatment-150428035837-conversion-gate01/95/now-arthritis-can-easily-curable-in-homeopathy-treatment-2-638.jpg?cb=1430193929

95

Presenting Symptoms and Signs

- Symmetric joint pain
- Swelling of small peripheral joints
- Morning joint stiffness of variable duration
- Other diffuse aching
- Fatigue, malaise, and depression may precede other symptoms by weeks or months

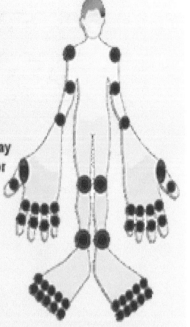

96

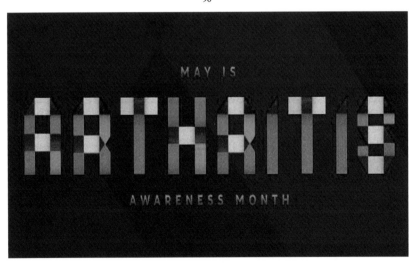

---

95 http://www.rheumatoid-arthritisdiet.com/images/Signs%20of%20Rheumatoid%20Arthritis.jpg

96 https://rheumatoidarthritis.net/wp-content/uploads/2014/05/20140507.jpg

97

What is Rheumatoid Disease?
also known as Rheumatoid Arthritis (RA)

RA is a progressive, destructive disease frequently leading to disability. It affects 1% of the population.

Immune cells attack joints & organs, including heart & lungs.

Symptoms like fatigue, joint pain, stiffness, swelling, & fever may be constant or flaring.

Almost 2/3 of patients have a 20% response or less to treatments. No cure is known.

U.S. spends a fraction on RA research of what is spent on rarer diseases with similar mortality rates.

more information at rheum4us.org
© 2012 Rheumatoid Patient Foundation

98

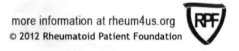

FACT #1: RHEUMATOID DISEASE IS NOT A TYPE OF ARTHRITIS.

IT IS A SYSTEMIC ILLNESS RELATED TO IMMUNE FUNCTION THAT CAN AFFECT ANY PART OF THE BODY INCLUDING LUNGS, HEART, EYES, SKIN AND JOINTS.

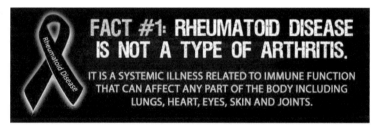

Disease

Rheumatoid ~~Arthritis~~

Arthritis is just one symptom.

#THE REAL RD
RHEUMATOID PATIENT FOUNDATION | RHEUM4US.ORG

---

[97] http://rheum4us.org/wp-content/uploads/2012/12/RA-info.jpg
[98] http://rawarrior.com/wp-content/uploads/2016/02/RD-FACTS-1.png

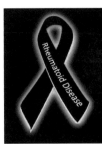

FACT #2: AVAILABLE TREATMENTS ARE NOT ADEQUATE

FOR MANY PEOPLE WITH MODERATE TO SEVERE RHEUMATOID DISEASE.

ABOUT 1/3
OF PEOPLE WITH RHEUMATOID DISEASE
DO NOT RESPOND
TO AVAILABLE BIOLOGICAL DISEASE MODIFYING DRUGS.

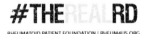

RHEUMATOID PATIENT FOUNDATION | RHEUM4US.ORG

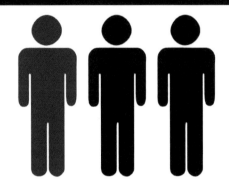

THE REAL RHEUMATOID DISEASE
FACT #3

RHEUMATOID DISEASE MANIFESTS ITSELF DIFFERENTLY IN EACH PERSON AND EVEN IN THE SAME PERSON OVER TIME.

#THEREALRD
RHEUMATOID PATIENT FOUNDATION | RHEUM4US.ORG

---

[99] http://rawarrior.com/wp-content/uploads/2016/02/RD-FACTS-2.png
[100] http://rawarrior.com/wp-content/uploads/2016/01/the-real-rheumatoid-disease-fact3-400x300.png

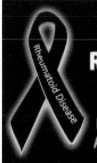

FACT #4: RESEARCH FOR RHEUMATOID DISEASE IS SEVERELY UNDERFUNDED IN THE U.S.

RHEUMTOID DISEASE RESEARCH RECEIVES ABOUT 1/12 THE AVERAGE PER-PATIENT FUNDING OF COMPARABLE DISEASES

AVERAGE YEARLY PER-PATIENT RESEARCH FUNDING

RHEUMATOID DISEASE
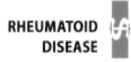

SIMILAR DISEASES
(LUPUS, DIABETES, MS)
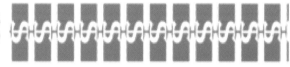

RHEUMATOID PATIENT FOUNDATION | RHEUM4US.ORG

Rheumatoid Awareness Day

February 2nd

Together we can do more!

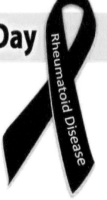

---

[101] http://rawarrior.com/wp-content/uploads/2016/01/RD-FACTS-4-400x298.png
[102] http://twibbon.s3.amazonaws.com/2013/22/92feb1e4-3bc1-4a7c-8a5f-e3a3596 a4855.jpg

21. Diabetes

Diabetes
Signs & Symptoms

*Polydypsia   *Marked irritability

*Polyuria   *Recurrence of bed wetting

*Polyphagia   *Drowsiness

*Loss of weight   *Malaise

*Loss of strength

Type 1: the onset of symptoms is sudden

Type 2: The onset of symptoms is slow & the cardinal
signs are less commonly seen.

104

Symptoms of Type 1 Diabetes

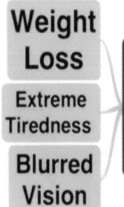

Weight Loss

Extreme Tiredness

Blurred Vision

Going To The Toilet More Frequently Especially At Night

Increased Thirst

Testing For Type 1 Diabetes Is Fast Painless And Only Takes A Few Seconds

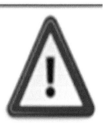

Do Not Ignore The Warning Signs See your Doctor As Soon As Possible

---

[103] https://image.slidesharecdn.com/diabetesadrenalinsufficiencythyroiddisease-nov-2007-140414054352-phpapp02/95/diabetes-adrenal-insufficiency-thyroid-disease-nov2007-7-638.jpg?cb=1397456032
[104] http://www.topdiabetestreatment.com/wp-content/uploads/2015/11/what-is-Type-1-Diabetes-Symptoms-treatment-cure.png

Warning Signs of Type 2 Diabetes

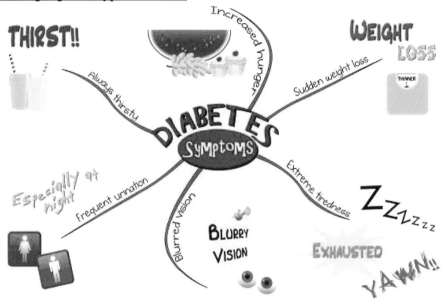

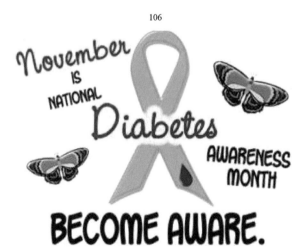

105 http://www.carefecthomecareservices.com/blog/wp-content/uploads/2014/05/
2014_05_22_Diabetes_WebRes.jpg
106 https://s-media-cache-ak0.pinimg.com/originals/81/7d/96/817d96c74cdc0aa1
bed3d428e6e1734a.jpg

CHAPTER 16. LIST OF CANCER TYPES[107]

Prior to researching, I never realized how many types of cancer we really deal with in life. I pray for all cancer patients to FULLY RECOVER and that the cancer NEVER RETURNS. *AMEN!*

Adrenal Cancer
Anal Cancer
Bile Duct Cancer
Bladder Cancer
Bone Cancer
Brain/CNS Tumors In Adults
Brain/CNS Tumors In Children
Breast Cancer
Breast Cancer In Men
Cancer in Adolescents
Cancer in Children
Cancer in Young Adults
Cancer of Unknown Primary
Castleman Disease
Cervical Cancer
Colon/Rectum Cancer
Endometrial Cancer
Esophagus Cancer
Ewing Family Of Tumors
Eye Cancer
Gallbladder Cancer
Gastrointestinal Carcinoid Tumors
Gastrointestinal Stromal Tumor (GIST)
Gestational Trophoblastic Disease
Hodgkin Disease
Kaposi Sarcoma
Kidney Cancer
Laryngeal and Hypopharyngeal Cancer
Leukemia
Leukemia - Acute Lymphocytic (ALL) in Adults
Leukemia - Acute Myeloid (AML)
Leukemia - Chronic Lymphocytic (CLL)
Leukemia - Chronic Myeloid (CML)
Leukemia - Chronic Myelomonocytic (CMML)
Leukemia in Children
Liver Cancer
Lung Cancer
Lung Cancer - Non-Small Cell
Lung Cancer - Small Cell
Lung Carcinoid Tumor
Lymphoma
Lymphoma of the Skin
Malignant Mesothelioma

---

[107] For more info.: http://www.cancer.org/cancer/showallcancertypes/index

Multiple Myeloma
Myelodysplastic Syndrome
Nasal Cavity and Paranasal Sinus Cancer
Nasopharyngeal Cancer
Neuroblastoma
Non-Hodgkin Lymphoma
Non-Hodgkin Lymphoma In Children
Oral Cavity and Oropharyngeal Cancer
Osteosarcoma
Ovarian Cancer
Pancreatic Cancer
Penile Cancer
Pituitary Tumors
Prostate Cancer
Retinoblastoma
Rhabdomyosarcoma
Salivary Gland Cancer
Sarcoma - Adult Soft Tissue Cancer
Skin Cancer
Skin Cancer - Basal and Squamous Cell
Skin Cancer - Melanoma
Skin Cancer - Merkel Cell
Small Intestine Cancer
Stomach Cancer
Testicular Cancer
Thymus Cancer
Thyroid Cancer
Uterine Sarcoma
Vaginal Cancer
Vulvar Cancer
Waldenstrom Macroglobulinemia
Wilms Tumor

List of Cancer Types

CHAPTER 17.   CANCER AND REMISSION[108]

What does it mean when cancer is in remission?

Complete remission means that there are no cancer cells found in the body based on tests, physical exams and scans of the body, according to WebMD. This can also be referred to as No Evidence of Disease, or NED.

Partial remission means that the cancer is still present, but the tumor has become smaller, or in the case of blood cancers, there is less cancer found throughout the body.

In both types of remission, this diagnosis does not mean that the cancer is cured, according to WebMD. Because it is impossible to tell whether or not all the cancer cells in the body are gone, the word "cured" is not commonly used with cancer. When cancer cells reappear, it typically happens within five years from the first diagnosis and treatment of cancer. When the cells reappear after an initial period of remission, this is called a recurrence of the cancer. While there is no way to predict the recurrence of cancer, there are steps that can be taken to minimize complications. Sticking to a schedule of recommended checkups is critical whether or not symptoms are present. Follow up care once remission is achieved most often includes regular blood work, physical exams and imaging tests.

---

[108] For more questions: https://www.reference.com/health/mean-cancer-remission-6c9ad22a86e47ef2?qo=cdpArticles

All Cancers
Lavender

Appendix Cancer
Amber

Bladder Cancer
Marigold/Blue/Purple

Brain Cancer
Grey

Breast Cancer
Pink

Carcinoid Cancer
Zebra Stripe

Cervical Cancer
Teal/White

Childhood Cancer
Gold

Colon Cancer
Dark Blue

Esophageal Cancer
Periwinkle

Gallbladder/Bile Duct
Cancer Kelly Green

Head & Neck Cancer
Burgundy/Ivory

Hodgkin's Lymphoma
Violet

Kidney Cancer
Orange

Leiomyosarcoma
Purple

Leukemia
Orange

Liver Cancer
Emerald Green

Lung Cancer
White

Lymphoma
Lime

Melanoma
Black

Multiple Myeloma
Burgundy

Ovarian Cancer
Teal

Pancreatic Cancer
Purple

Prostate Cancer
Light Blue

Sarcoma/Bone Cancer
Yellow

Stomach Cancer
Periwinkle

Testicular Cancer
Orchid

Thyroid Cancer
Teal/Pink/Blue

Uterine Cancer
Peach

Honors Caregivers
Plum

Click here for a printable chart of
**CANCER AWARENESS
RIBBON COLORS**

---

[109] https://s-media-cache-ak0.pinimg.com/originals/2d/83/4d/2d834dd78fa4bc3ad1
ea3ea17e4afd9c.png

CHAPTER 19.   HURRICANE MATTHEW & THE
BLESSINGS THAT FOLLOWED

In October 2016, Hurricane Matthew affected a number of people, including those in my hometown in South Carolina. So many have lost their lives and homes due to this enormous and deadly storm. And here in the South, poor weather conditions have always affected our area. It's also a fact that we get a great deal of rain which possibly leads to floods and other hazardous conditions. The importance of keeping your eyes and ears open for updates on the weather is always imperative.

My deepest condolences go out to all who were impacted and those who didn't make it through this horrific hurricane. God bless each and every family member. *Amen.*

A BLESSING

Posted on FB – 10/5/16

**A Prayer for Those Threatened by the Effects
of Hurricane Matthew**

Lord,

We Pray for ALL those threatened by the effects of Hurricane Matthew. Please be with them during this difficult and scary time. We pray for protection, covering and comfort through all the loss. Please give us strength to come together as a community to help those who are in great need as a result of the destruction of this storm. In Jesus Name. Amen!!!

It was fortunate that we only went without electricity, but kept our lives. But at the same time, we were unfortunate to not have owned a generator. So, after a few days without electricity, my brother-in-law stopped by to drop off his electric generator. And oh what a relief it was to have such a beautiful blessing on our doorstep. My husband and I were so excited that I had to share this wonderful blessing on Facebook with all of my family and friends:

A BLESSING

Posted on FB – 10/9/16

My brother-in-law Lorenzo is one special guy. Through the storm the man provided us with a generator to help with the lack of electricity in our home. Hurricane Matthew had us with no electricity for the past 40 hours straight. May God bless Lorenzo in every joyous way possible.
Thanks again brother-in-law. *Amen.*

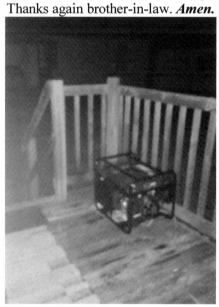

This was such a loving and surprising thought on his part. God is always on time.

Since the electrical outage began on October 7 and my brother-in-law provided an electric generator on October 9, we were still praying for normal electricity by Momma's birthday on October 15.

Michelle & William
10/9/16

It was Sunday, the Lord's day, and attending morning church was the way the family enjoyed their day. But this Sunday for us in South Carolina, will never be forgotten.

That's when Hurricane Matthew decided to pay us a naughty visit. I was so concerned and worried about my husband and brother-in-law having to travel in this dangerous weather. But in order to operate the new generator, the need for gas was essential. Due to the poor weather conditions, almost all of the stores in and around town were closed. And if one was found open, the pumps were inoperable. The telephone lines were down, cell phones weren't working and, sadly, I was home alone with no one to talk to. The guys were gone for several hours and I didn't know what to do or think. But as soon as my cell phone was up and running, I gave them a call, but to no avail. I guess things weren't working okay on their end either.

A little while later, though I was still unable to make calls, texting somehow seemed to work. So the next people I texted was my niece Michelle and her husband William. By this time, I was crying ecstatically and needed someone to just listen first and then give me their suggestions. I needed someone desperately to talk to, even if it was only for a little while. I think I was looking for some sort of reassurance 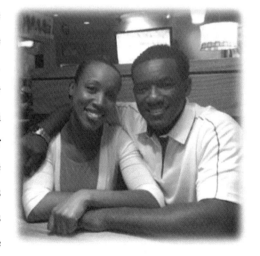 or comfort so that I would feel at ease while the guys were away.

So, at 12:21 p.m., I sent a text message to both Michelle and William and asked if they would pray for us. Their responses were quick, precise and right to the point. Both of you were there, in good faith, in true family love and in prayer.

SHIRLEY'S TEXT MESSAGE:

PLEASE SAY A LITTLE PRAYER FOR US. WE'VE BEEN W/O ELECTRIC FOR 32 HRS. NOW DUE 2 HURRICANE MATTHEW. LORENZO CAME BY W/ HIS NEW GENERATOR BUT HAVE 2 GET SOME GAS 2 GET IT STARTED. HE & ED R WORKING ON THAT RIGHT NOW. WISH US LUCK. THANK U & GOD BLESS. SHIRLEY & ED

***

WILLIAM'S RESPONSE AT 12:22 PM:

Praying for you, God bless

MICHELLE'S RESPONSE AT 12:26 PM:

*Father God, may you grant traveling mercies to Lorenzo and Ed as they go out for gas for the generator. Father God we pray that you keep Aunt Shirley, Ed and Lorenzo safe and out of harm's way. Father, we ask that you please quiet the storm. Heavenly Father we ask that you bring light to their moment of darkness. We love you Father. In Jesus' name we pray, **Amen.***

MICHELLE'S RESPONSE AT 12:33 PM

He is always with us -- through our trials and triumphs. Continue to pray to Him for everything. Love you.

***

Shortly later, I received a telephone call from my husband indicating that he and my brother-in-law were on their way back home. He explained how they were able to get the gas for the generator but had to travel to the South of the Border to

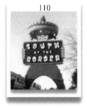

110

[110] https://scontent-iad3-1.xx.fbcdn.net/v/t1.0-0/s480x480/16681940_252349688508
204_6995945086788177536_n.jpg?oh=e78f1b109aaf69742adaae83e41f5363&oe=59287
02B

retrieve it. South of the Border is an attraction on Interstate 95 and US Highway 301/501 in Dillon, South Carolina, just south of Rowland, North Carolina. It is so named because it is just south of the border between North Carolina and South Carolina and is tongue-in-cheek themed in faux Mexican style. The rest area contains restaurants, gas stations, and a motel, and truck stop as well as a small dilapidated amusement park with no operating rides but a mini golf course still in commission, shopping and fireworks stores. Its mascot is Pedro, a caricature of a Mexican bandido.[111]

I was happy and sad at the same time; happy that they were able to get the gas, but sad that they were frustrated and exhausted from traveling for over five hours to do so. But returning home safely was so much more important to me than anything. I believe that through Michelle and William's prayers, the safety of our family was assured. Thank you Lord for another blessing. *Amen.*

A BLESSING

Posted on FB – 10/11/16

Out and about this beautiful Tuesday. Enjoying this day with hubby and brother-in-law. Still praying for electricity but not complaining at all. There are so many with less. I'm feeling thankful and blessed for another day. GOD BLESS US ALL, ESPECIALLY THE ONES WHO HAVE LESS. AMEN!!!

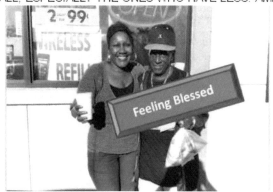

---

[111] See more: https://en.wikipedia.org/wiki/South_of_the_Border_(attraction)

Well, it's Momma's birthday and it's also the eighth day without normal electricity. But the first thing on my list this morning was to post a Happy Birthday tribute on Facebook to show Momma some love.

Posted on FB – 10/15/16

LOVING AND MISSING MOM ON HER SPECIAL DAY!
HAPPY BIRTHDAY - RIP!

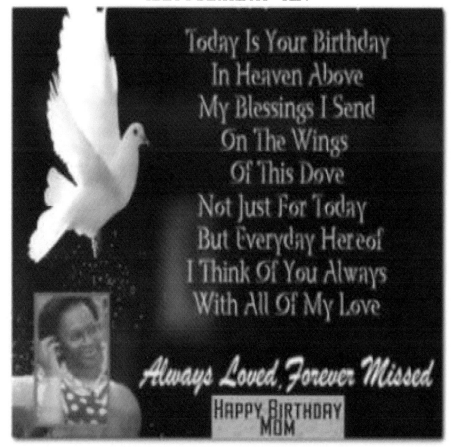

And only less than two hours after posting Momma's birthday message, the electricity was back on. I couldn't wait to return to Facebook to post this miraculous event and to show folks how God mysteriously performs his work. How He and my mother were both watching over us that very day. *Amen.*

228

AND GOD SAID... LET THERE BE LIGHT...

OH YES, THE ELECTRICITY JUST CAME BACK ON. I KNEW YOU WERE WATCHING OVER US MOM. IT TOOK YOUR SPECIAL BIRTHDAY TO MAKE OUR DAY COME ALIVE!!! THANK YOU. AMEN.

Thanksgiving Eve Holiday Photo

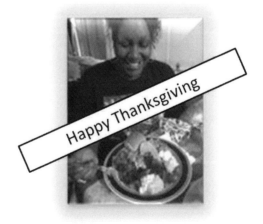

I consider this the meal of all times. This is the family holiday I've been waiting for. Thank you Lord. *Amen.*

Brother-in-law Lorenzo
December 2016

My brother-in-law Lorenzo has been thinking about relocating to South Carolina for some time now. But once his decision was confirmed, he was presented with a poem that I wrote several years earlier. Actually, I didn't know who this poem was really meant for. I was just writing what I was actually feeling at that time. But now I know. It was meant for my brother-in-law Lorenzo. *Amen.*

Special Neighbor

Our tears represent the rain
Our laughter represents the sun
Our sadness represents the moon
And our strange sense of humor represents the stars

The world at large in our vulnerable minds
Wrapped in the center of our very souls
When we gaze at the above, we may call
For love and determination for us all

We know our weaknesses as well as our strengths
We will not allow ourselves to be tense
We fear what we don't know
And we beg for forgiveness as the minutes flow

Let us pray for the better things in life
Let us teach for the higher high
Let us smell the fruits of labor
God will send us a very special neighbor

Shirley Valentine

Knowing that family is not so far away after all, is my idea of happy future events together. We have been blessed once again in our journey of life.

It may sound a bit selfish but who cares; it's family and that's all that matters. Now I know the true meaning of a "Special Neighbor." *Amen.*

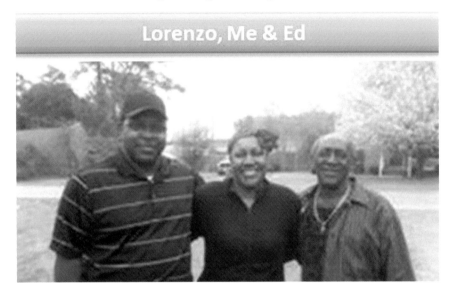

In the past, we've shared some incredible times in Coney Island together. Acting like young love-struck teenagers as we took photos on this beautiful summer day. Our husbands were gracious enough to take us on a surprise getaway trip and spoil us rotten in the process. Thanks. You guys are the best. *God bless.*

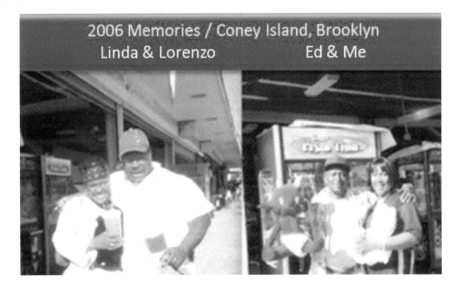

A BLESSING

Early Holiday Greetings

Early Holiday Greetings from my friendly neighbors the Jackson Family, "Home Grown Collard Greens". Have to enjoy these for the Holidays. God Bless and Amen!

Thank You For...

Thank You for delicious yummies
To fill our hungry, grateful tummies.
For other things we're thinking of
And for Your everlasting love,
For all the blessings that You bring,
Thank you God, for everything.

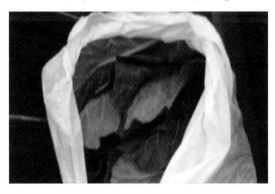

CHAPTER 20. FACEBOOK

A. FAMILY & FRIENDS / SIDEKICKS

One thing about Facebook is that everybody has family and friends. But to have a special sidekick is something totally different. I use the term genuinely because in my case, it demonstrates a partnership of crazy loyalty that sometimes, doesn't have to really make sense — as long as someone has got your back. *Amen.*

My nieces Leslie and Kashana, and Deborah's daughter Tahisha are third cousins and also my sidekicks on and off of Facebook. These three ladies have shown me mucho love through my illness and recently, Facebook is how we've been staying in touch. *Amen.*

Over the past few years, these ladies have shared so many beautiful and exciting moments together and have become even closer than ever. My family knows how important it is for me to see their happy smiles and to be informed of their crazy and exciting activities. LOL. Our family believes in family first, and that's how we maintain our strength. And although these ladies may have their hands full with their household and work, occasionally they have to make time just for themselves. Sharing special moments with family on girls'

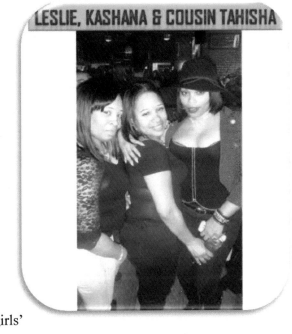

LESLIE, KASHANA & COUSIN TAHISHA

night out, is how my family relishes themselves. I love my family. *Amen.*

233

Shanda is Cousin Bill's granddaughter, and she has been involved with the recovery of my health on Facebook as well. I haven't had the opportunity to see my family for quite some time now. But lately, Cousin Shanda has shown love and dedication just by saying "hello" and "how are you?" Words like these mean a lot more than people think. Keeping up with the growth and communication of our family functions was a great help for my recovery. *Amen!*

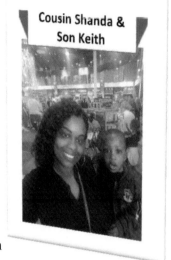

Cousin Shanda & Son Keith

With all the excitement surrounding them, Cousin Shanda's adorable and handsome son Keith is surprised as he accompanies his mom on a beautiful day at the mall. How blessed can one person be to have such a beautiful family! *Amen.*

These fine gentlemen, Dion and Shawn, are Aunt Sara's two handsome sons and Big Naheen's first cousins. Whenever I was down and out, these guys would give me their hearts to wear on my sleeves. Cousin Shawn kept my spirits up by displaying Facebook videos of cooking delicious meals for their mom as well as handling other household matters. When Aunt Sara's birthday or any other unique event occurred, the family would celebrate by sharing special dinners and lots of prayers. Cousin Dion and I would share and discuss prayer posts with one another on Facebook. We would also laugh about the good times we all shared in the past. *Amen.*

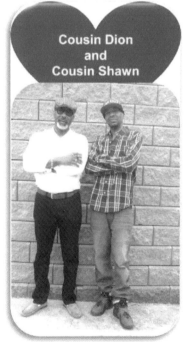

Cousin Dion and Cousin Shawn

Thanks again cousins for showing me the love I needed by sharing your pics, videos and telephone calls. You both have made my life more appreciative than ever. May you continue to share your loving ways with others. *Amen.*

These attractive and great-looking people are Cousin Bill's grandchildren and my cousins. Through my illness, they have managed to encourage me with

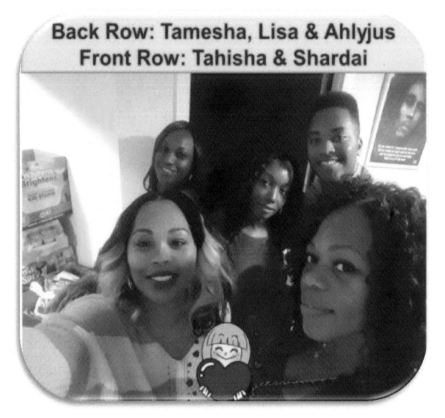

prayers which helped me achieve a successful recovery. They continuously share pics, videos and prayers on Facebook. May God bless my beautiful family. *Amen.*

Yvette is Uncle Vince's granddaughter and my cousin. This fine brown frame has got it going on, and there's no stopping her. Cousin Yvette continues to shine as she sports her sexy and glowing looks for the world to see. *Amen cuz.* You have in the past, and still do, show great love for me on and off of Facebook. I love seeing my family as they share so many loving pics of family and friends. And, although we may live so many miles apart, I'm grateful to have a cousin who makes me feel like I'm her next door neighbor. ***Amen.***

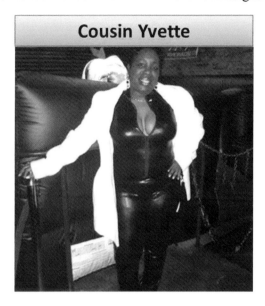

Cousin Yvette

Pamela is also Uncle Vince's granddaughter, as well as the younger sister of Yvette. Cousin Pamela shares a pic of herself as she strolls down memory lane. LOL. My cousin looks absolutely marvelous and I'm very proud to have her in my life. As family, she has always showed me love and support on and off of Facebook. My cousin is very thoughtful when sharing precious pics and videos of family and

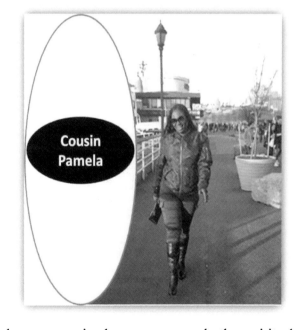

Cousin Pamela

friends. I especially love it when my cousin shares prayers and other spiritual quotes on Facebook as well. Our prayers of me getting better have graciously

236

been answered and may you continue to keep the spirits of others up — for your soul is real cuzzo. I will always love and respect my beautiful cousin. *Amen.*

My nieces are always on time when it comes down to loyalty and dedication on and off of Facebook. They continue to show their aunt love and respect by staying in touch and keeping me apprised of any special events pertaining to my grandniece and grandnephews. Being my special sidekicks has given me the strength in my recovering process.

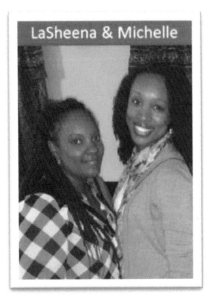

LaSheena & Michelle

To LaSheena & Michelle: Thank you so much ladies for showing the love and understanding that Momma gave to all her grandchildren. You both have been understanding and patient during my illness and I will never forget the loyalty you've shown throughout. May God bless you both. *Amen.*

Wanda is the older sister of my deceased girlfriend, Sherrell, and I'm so glad I had the opportunity to meet her. Wanda has been there for me, even after Sherrell's sudden demise. Being my special sidekick in sharing spiritual and motivational posts on Facebook, has been a tremendous blessing to me. We've also shared video chat on Facebook as well.

To Wanda: Thank you Wanda for being the beautiful sister Sherrell always spoke fondly of. I'm especially grateful to you for being a loving and dedicated person who stood by her sister's side while she went through her fight with lung cancer. I have known you for some time now, and I hope and pray that our friendship will continue to be blessed. In Jesus Name. *Amen.*

Wanda & Sister Sherrell

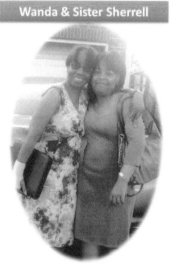

Wanda

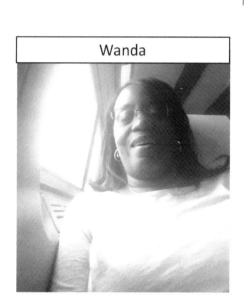

Linda is my family, friend and sidekick on and off of Facebook. Although we may not be related by blood, she has been, and still is, the long-time soulmate of my nephew, Steven Jr.

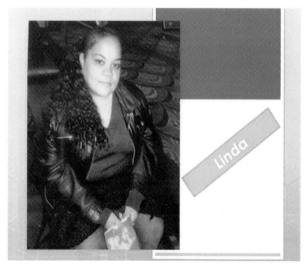

Linda

To Linda: You've been there for me during the lowest point of my life and I truly respect you for that. Your compassion for others is a blessing which I know caught the attention of my nephew. You've taken the time to share positive and inspirational quotes, video chat and world news on Facebook with me. Thank you so much for being yourself as well as being good to my nephew, as he is to you. May God bless you both. *Amen.*

I met Evette through her cousin, Big Naheen, in 1979, but out of respect for elders, she would always address us as Uncle Junior and Aunt Shirley. Cousin Evette is the daughter of Aunt Linda as well as the oldest of her other two siblings.

Cousin Evette and her husband William have been together since December 2006, and after almost three years together, they realized that they were actually soulmates. So, on September 2009, their hearts were intertwined into one union. God has given my niece the man she has always dreamed of. *Amen.*

William dotes on his beautiful wife, and I love seeing it all on Facebook. Posting joys of birthdays, anniversaries, and other holidays were shared with others. This young lady gets served right up when her husband brings home the bacon, flowers, candy, hugs and a whole lot more. *Amen.*

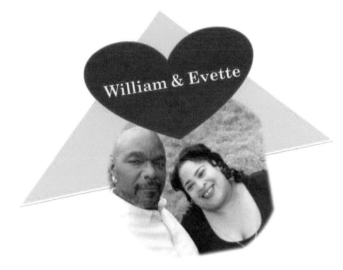

Cousin Evette also has two handsome and amazing sons, Mar'Ques the youngest, and Shahiem the oldest, and they truly adore their mother.

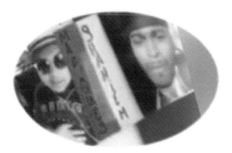

On several occasions, Cousin Evette would post daily pics on Facebook in regards to the day of the week. Example: Marvelous Monday; Thirsty Tuesday; Wacky Wednesday; Thankful Thursday; and Fabulous Friday. She would also add a few pics of herself, dressed in her own creative style while also presenting positive quotes on Facebook to family and friends. *Amen.*

Cousin Evette is employed as a school bus driver, and not just any bus driver. She is an active participant in providing safe travels for the children as well as getting involved in their holiday spirits. She decorates her school bus on special occasions, interacts with the children by sharing jokes, games and anything positive that would uplift their spirits. Cousin Evette is remarkable in showing others the beauty of the world. She cares a great deal for children and have, for many, many years.

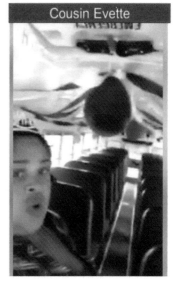
Cousin Evette

In November 2016, Cousin Evette celebrated the Thanksgiving Holiday as well as her birthday and other birthdays on the bus. According to Cousin Evette, on this holiday, this was Ms. Red's November Thanksgiving Birthday Holiday and Decorations. A beautiful and exciting day was shared with Evette and the children. *Amen.*

Cousin Evette continues to create funny and hilarious Facebook posts which I continue to enjoy until this day.

To Cousin Evette: Thank you for giving me the excitement I needed in my life in order to get better. You have been one of the sweetest sidekicks I know. May God bless you and your family always.

Renarda and I met when I moved to Andrews, South Carolina. She and I were both associated with the same apartment complex and shared many great times together. One of our most precious moments was when her daughter Arianna was born. This little sweetheart was born on the same day that Ed and I moved into our home. Arianna's father Marvin, helped us with the move, and by the end of the day, was called to go to the hospital to be there for the birth of his baby girl. God bless and thanks for being my true special sidekick on and off of Facebook!

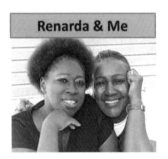

A very special neighbor came by to visit me for the day. Thank you God for bringing good friends into my life. Amen!

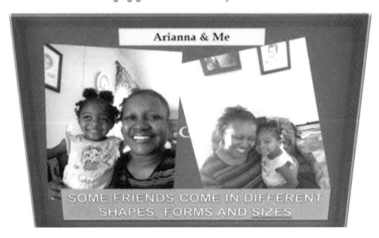

Last, but not least, my buddy and sidekick on and off of Facebook — Keith. We have been past co-workers as well as friends since January, 2007. You, along with other co-workers (Adrienne, Virginia, Ann Marie and others) have been involved with the recovery of my illness. Once you were informed, you got involved immediately and removed some of my pain by sharing prayers, words of encouragement quotes and other inspirational quotes on Facebook, among other things.

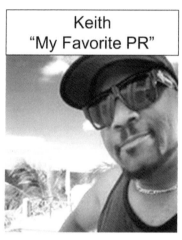

Keith
"My Favorite PR"

Over the years, our friendships have grown even stronger, and today, we still continue to maintain relationships on Facebook. I truly believe that our relationships have withstood the test of time because true friendship comes straight from the heart and not the pocket(book)! Thanks again sidekicks — together with prayer, we were able to overcome! *Amen.*

B. AWARENESS

Unfortunately, many people insist on utilizing Facebook as a tool for sharing negative behavior. It amazes me how people can go on and on about Facebook and all the negativity that goes along with it. But then, they continue to use it.

In my opinion, Facebook itself was never the problem — it's only the people who decide to post and say negative things. They're the ones with the problem. Guess what ... if you only post positive things and keep a positive attitude or just say nothing at all, then you're ok. If you see the same type of posts, use the same tactic. End of Story! As my Cousin Tahisha would say:

Cousin Tahisha

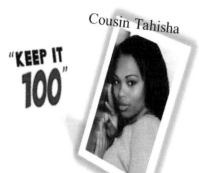

I truly believe that Facebook does not intend to be used in any negative, malicious or derogatory manner.

We have to take note that certain things are posted about individuals who aren't even on Facebook. So, don't think because you don't have an account in Facebook, nothing is being said about you. Positive or negative, it doesn't make a difference — gossip spreads anyway. Unaware of what the future may hold, it's always best to take into consideration, that what we post today can affect our children of tomorrow. Therefore, think wisely because one thing we can't stop, and that's progress! Facebook is a fast-growing website that should be used in a positive manner. As a result, you can utilize it wisely, or unwisely — the decision is yours to make.

C. WHAT FACEBOOK HAS TAUGHT ME

THIS BOOK SHOWS THE MANY POSITIVE WAYS FACEBOOK CAN BE UTILIZED, AND I RESPECTFULLY HOPE OTHERS FOLLOW SIMILAR BEHAVIOR. AMEN.

Do not get involved too deeply with Facebook unless you are doing positive things with it. There is an abundance of negative behavior with increasingly uncountable 'Likes' and not enough 'Likes' for more positive behavior. This positive, of course, should always include praises to our Lord. I've never claimed to be a Saint and I'm not even close to being one, but I will take time to praise His name and try my very best to live by His ways. *Amen.*

My experience on Facebook while dealing with cancer was a spiritual experience for me. It may sound a little crazy to you — you're probably saying "How in the world can Facebook be a spiritual experience for you?" Well, it was easy, due to the fact that I couldn't get around like I wanted to, and with much of my family residing outside of South Carolina, Facebook actually brought us closer together.

Facebook also allows me to get more in touch with God. Periodically posting spiritual quotes, inspirational quotes, words of wisdom and other quotes did amazing things. It makes me so abundantly happy when family and friends admire and want to share positivity. This process makes me feel extremely loved and God's blessings will continue to flow throughout Facebook if I can help it. This is God's work — speaking positive thoughts and prayers through social media.

I truly believe that God has showed me the way of getting more involved with Facebook. The new way of reaching out to your family and friends is through social media. What other way could I have actually shared pics and videos?

On June 17, 2016, I believe God wanted me to spend less time on Facebook and more time on improving myself. So I decided to send out this post to all my family and friends:

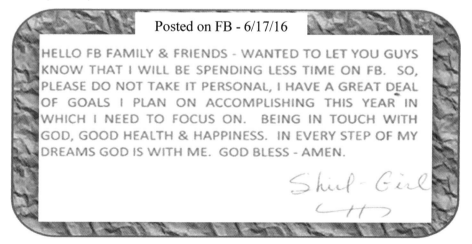

Posted on FB - 6/17/16

HELLO FB FAMILY & FRIENDS - WANTED TO LET YOU GUYS KNOW THAT I WILL BE SPENDING LESS TIME ON FB. SO, PLEASE DO NOT TAKE IT PERSONAL, I HAVE A GREAT DEAL OF GOALS I PLAN ON ACCOMPLISHING THIS YEAR IN WHICH I NEED TO FOCUS ON. BEING IN TOUCH WITH GOD, GOOD HEALTH & HAPPINESS. IN EVERY STEP OF MY DREAMS GOD IS WITH ME. GOD BLESS - AMEN.

Shief-Girl

THAT'S RIGHT! TIME TO SPEND MORE TIME ON ME & MY GOALS...

Usually, I would copy, share and post morning prayers. However, in late June, I began re-creating my own morning prayer posts — posting every other day or so. At times, I would add in a cartoon character such as Tweety Bird or Mickey Mouse, a "good morning" address and the word-of-the-day. All other information have been copied and shared with others on Facebook, keeping in mind, all posts are a reflection of the Lord's work. *AMEN.*

SOME OF MY INSPIRATIONAL POSTS:

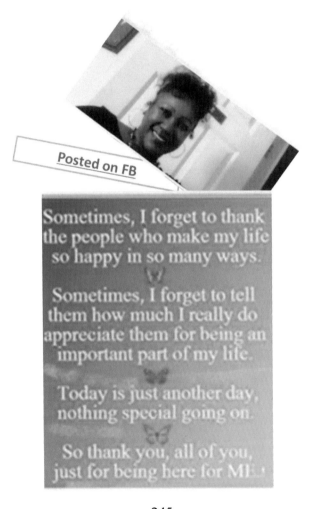

Posted on FB

Sometimes, I forget to thank the people who make my life so happy in so many ways.

Sometimes, I forget to tell them how much I really do appreciate them for being an important part of my life.

Today is just another day, nothing special going on.

So thank you, all of you, just for being here for ME.

Good Morning FB Family & Friends

IT'S THURSDAY
JUNE 23, 2016

Thank you God for waking me up this morning.
Thank you God for allowing me to see another day.
Thank you God for keeping my family safe.

AND, IF YOU'RE HAPPY GOD WOKE YOU UP
THIS BEAUTIFUL MORNING, SAY "AMEN"

AMEN

SValentine/6-23-16

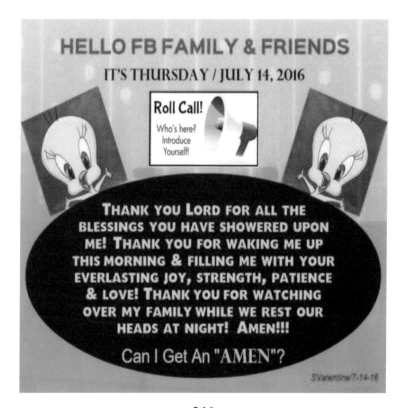

HELLO FB FAMILY & FRIENDS
IT'S FRIDAY / JULY 15, 2016

HAVE A BEAUTIFUL & BLESSED WEEKEND

WE ALL NEED JESUS

A Prayer for Strength

Our Father,
Sometimes the cares of the day
seem to multiply, while the
blessings fade so quickly.
Our bodies grow tired
and our minds even more tired.
Jesus, help us.
Give us the strength You've promised
in Your Word.
Give us the power
to take the next step.
Give us your grace...
for we know that in our weaknesses
YOUR STRENGTH is revealed.
May we receive it today.
Amen.

dlwojo.com

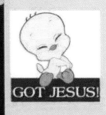

GOT JESUS!

GOD BLESS

Can I Get An "AMEN"?

SValentine/7-15-16

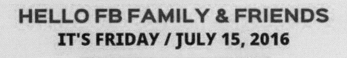

HELLO FB FAMILY & FRIENDS

It's Thursday / July 21, 2016

CONTENTMENT

DEAR GLORIOUS FATHER,

I PRAY THAT I WILL STAY FOCUSED ON
YOU TODAY. I PRAY THAT YOU WILL
CONSTANTLY REMIND ME TO BE CONTENT
IN ALL OF MY CIRCUMSTANCES. I PRAY
THAT YOU WILL FILL ME UP THAT I MAY
BE JOYFUL ALL DAY, EVEN IF STRESS
CREEPS IN. I KNOW THAT THROUGH MY
CONTENTMENT, YOU WILL BE GLORIFIED.
I WANT TO HONOR YOU, FATHER, IN
ALL THAT I DO. I PRAISE YOUR HOLY
NAME! AMEN!!!

If You Believe, Type **'AMEN'**

SValentine/7-21-16

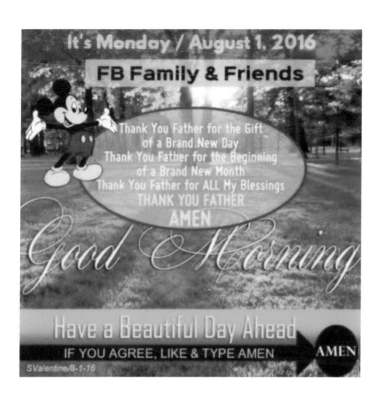

It's Monday / August 1, 2016

FB Family & Friends

Thank You Father for the Gift
of a Brand New Day
Thank You Father for the Beginning
of a Brand New Month
Thank You Father for ALL My Blessings
THANK YOU FATHER
AMEN

Good Morning

Have a Beautiful Day Ahead

IF YOU AGREE, LIKE & TYPE AMEN   AMEN

SValentine/8-1-16

HELLO FB FAMILY & FRIENDS
It's Friday / August 5, 2016

EARLY MORNING PRAYER

Dear LORD,

I THANK YOU for the Grace of
being alive this morning; I
THANK YOU for the sleep that
has refreshed me; I THANK
YOU for the chance to make a
new beginning. AMEN

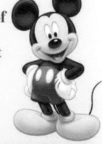

If You Agree, Type "AMEN"

AMEN

SValentine/8-5-16

GOOD MORNING FACEBOOK
FAMILY & FRIENDS
HELLO SATURDAY & SUNDAY

A morning prayer
There are so many things I take for granted.
May I not ignore them today.
Just for today, help me, God, to remember that my
life is a gift, that my health is a blessing, that this
new day is filled with awesome potential, that I
have the capacity to bring something wholly new
and unique and good into this world.
Just for today, help me, God, to remember to be
kind and patient to the people who love me, and to
those who work with me too. Teach me to see all
the beauty that I so often ignore, and to listen to the
silent longing of my own soul.
Just for today, help me, God, to remember You.
Let this be a good day, God, full of joy and love.
Amen.
Read, Love and Learn
facebook.com/readloveandlearn

"HAVE
A
SAFE
AND
BLESSED
WEEKEND"

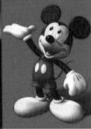

Can I Get An AMEN? AMEN

SValentine/8-13-16&8-14-16

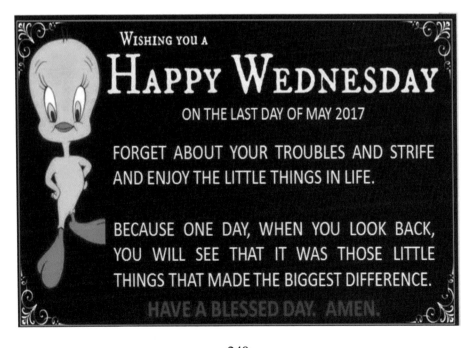

WISHING YOU A

HAPPY WEDNESDAY
ON THE LAST DAY OF MAY 2017

FORGET ABOUT YOUR TROUBLES AND STRIFE
AND ENJOY THE LITTLE THINGS IN LIFE.

BECAUSE ONE DAY, WHEN YOU LOOK BACK,
YOU WILL SEE THAT IT WAS THOSE LITTLE
THINGS THAT MADE THE BIGGEST DIFFERENCE.

HAVE A BLESSED DAY. AMEN.

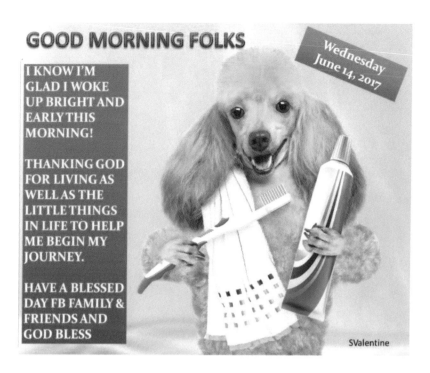

Anniversary and Birthday Posts

Happy Birthday Naheen! Loved and never forgotten. Miss you Man. Love Always, Shirley!!! Amen.

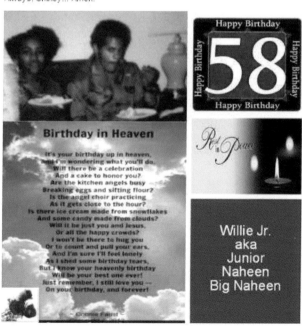

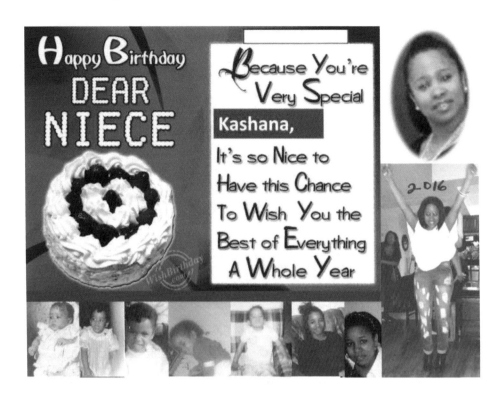

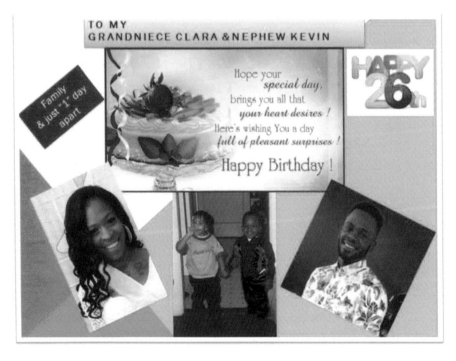

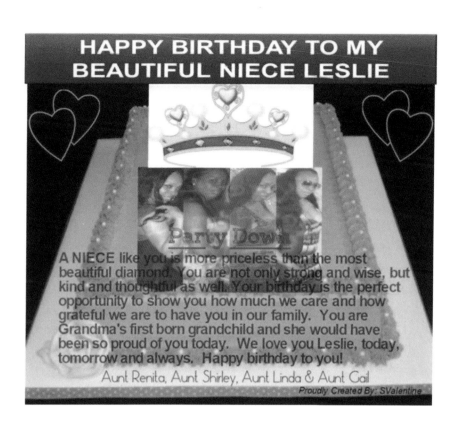

HAPPY BIRTHDAY TO MY BEAUTIFUL NIECE LESLIE

Party Down

A NIECE like you is more priceless than the most beautiful diamond. You are not only strong and wise, but kind and thoughtful as well. Your birthday is the perfect opportunity to show you how much we care and how grateful we are to have you in our family. You are Grandma's first born grandchild and she would have been so proud of you today. We love you Leslie, today, tomorrow and always. Happy birthday to you!

Aunt Renita, Aunt Shirley, Aunt Linda & Aunt Gail

Proudly Created By: SValentine

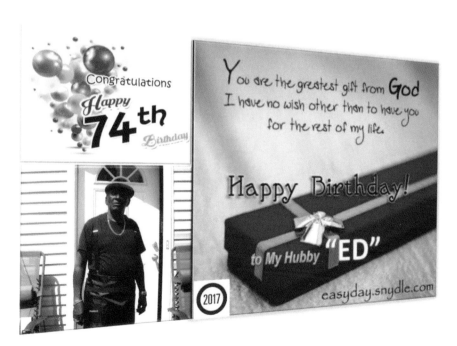

Congratulations

Happy **74th** *Birthday*

You are the greatest gift from God I have no wish other than to have you for the rest of my life.

Happy Birthday!

to My Hubby "ED"

2017

easyday.snydle.com

BIRTHDAY PRAYER

Thank you, God, for giving me another year of life.
Thank you for all the people who remembered me today
by sending cards, and letters, gifts and good wishes.

Thank you for all the experience of this past year;
for times of success which will always be happy memories,
for times of failure which reminded me of my own
weakness and of my need for you,
for times of joy when the sun was shining,
for times of sadness which drove me to you.

Forgive me
for the hours I wasted,
for the chances I failed to take,
for the opportunities I missed this past year.
Help me in the days ahead to make this the best year yet,
and through it to bring good credit to myself,
happiness and pride to my loved ones,
and joy to you. Amen.

A Prayer Against Cancer Post

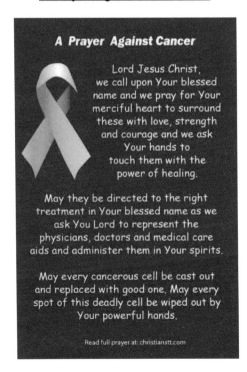

A Prayer Against Cancer

Lord Jesus Christ,
we call upon Your blessed
name and we pray for Your
merciful heart to surround
these with love, strength
and courage and we ask
Your hands to
touch them with the
power of healing.

May they be directed to the right
treatment in Your blessed name as we
ask You Lord to represent the
physicians, doctors and medical care
aids and administer them in Your spirits.

May every cancerous cell be cast out
and replaced with good one. May every
spot of this deadly cell be wiped out by
Your powerful hands.

Read full prayer at: christianstt.com

D. GOFUNDME | FACEBOOK

Fortunately, Facebook provides a link to the popular GoFundMe fundraising website.   Although I haven't created a GoFundMe account of my own, I've proudly made numerous donations to worthy causes.   GoFundMe allows you to create a campaign for you or someone else to receive donations in support of a particular cause. Money can be raised for many different causes and situations:

> homelessness; low income families; inventions; doctor bills; heroes; benevolent association; household bills; lost property; low income schools; battered women; mistreated animals; campaigns; and many more...

You never know when you or someone you love may need support or help. Helping others is the most heroic and gratifying experiences in life. *Amen.*
https://www.facebook.com/gofundme/

The easiest way to raise money online.[113]

There are no deadlines or goal requirements, and you get to keep every donation you receive.

All of our campaigns are mobile friendly, and you can even manage your campaign on-the-go with the GoFundMe Mobile App.[114, 115]

---

[113] http://www.Gofundme.com/contact
[114] Follow GoFundMe on Twitter: https://twitter.com/gofundme
[115] Follow GoFundMe on Instagram: https://www.instagram.com/gofundme/

What a difference it made in my life to share morning prayers with others via Facebook. Just one 'Like' would make my day. I also decided to write this book on overcoming cancer. Thank you Lord — you have been so good to me. *Amen.*

ALWAYS

REMEMBER TO

UTILIZE

FACEBOOK AS A

TOOL FOR

POSITIVE

PURPOSES

ONLY.

AMEN.

SPECIAL SHOUT-OUT & THANKS TO ALL MY FACEBOOK FAMILY & FRIENDS

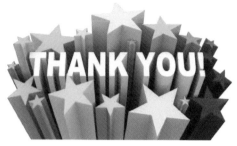

ADRIENNE, AHLYJUS, ANGELA, ANN MARIE, ARLENE, AUDREY, BARBARA, BILL, BRENDA, BRIAN, CARL, CECIL (RIP), CHARLENE, CHARLES, CHENNEL, CLARA, CYNTHIA, DEBBIE, DEBORAH, DEE, DELORES, DIANE, DION, ED, EDITH, ELAINE, EULA, EVETTE, GAIL, GREGORY, GWEN, IBRAHIM, JACKIE, JEFFREY, JENNIFER, JERRY, JOHN, KAREN, KASHANA, KEISHA, KEITH, KELVIN, KENDRA, KENNETH, KEVIN, KIMMIE (RIP), KRISTINA, LASHEENA, LAURA, LAVERN, LEROY, LESLIE, LEWANDA, LINDA, LISA, LIZA, LIZZY, LORENZO, LUIS, MAGGIE, MAMITA, MAR'QUES, MARVIN, MATILDE, MATTHEW, MERLYN, MICHAEL, MICHELLE, MIKE, MONICA, NAHDREAMS, NAQUAN, NATALIE, ORIN, PAM, PAMELA, PATRICIA, PATRICE, PETE, RAMEL, RANDY, RENARDA, RENITA, RICK, ROBERT, SAL, SARA, SHAHEEM, SHAHIEM, SHAKEERA, SHANDA, SHANIQUE, SHARDAI, SHARESE, SHAWN, STEVE, STEVEN, SYLVIA, TAHISHA, TAMESHA, TERESA, TERRY, TIFFANY, TINA, TONIO, TONY, TYRONE, UNIQUE, VAUGHN, VERONICA, VIRGINIA, WANDA, WAUNDELL, WILL, WILLIAM, YONNIE, YVETTE, YVONNE AND SO MANY MORE WONDERFUL PEOPLE!

MY FAVORITE PR — THANKS FOR ALL OF YOUR INSPIRATION, SUPPORT, PRAYERS, LOYALTY AND DEDICATION IN HELPING A FRIEND IN NEED. I WILL FOREVER BE GRATEFUL TO YOU.

IN LOVING MEMORY
May 2017

Girlfriend Kimmie:

> I'm so glad we were able to enjoy a nice long conversation
> via video chat in Facebook. I still remember your laugh and
> wonderful sense of humor. Rest in Peace my long-time
> friend. You will be greatly missed.
> Love always, Shirley & Family

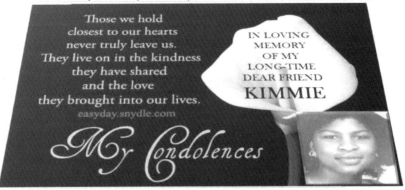

Former Co-Worker and Friend Cecil:

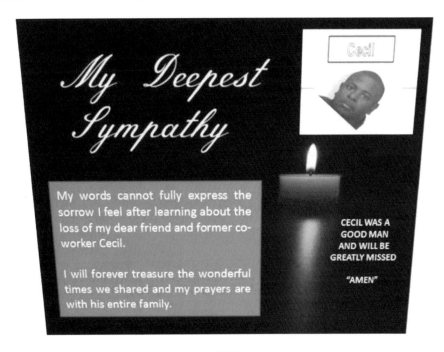

ST. JOHN 15:7

"IF YE ABIDE IN ME, AND MY WORDS ABIDE IN YOU, YE SHALL ASK WHAT YE WILL, AND IT SHALL BE DONE UNTO YOU!"

AMEN.
THANK YOU GOD
WITHOUT YOU THERE WOULD BE NO ME!

CPSIA information can be obtained at www.ICGtesting.com
Printed in the USA
LVIW01n1623140518
576896LV00026B/366